Tendon Transfers in the Foot and Ankle

Guest Editors

CHRISTOPHER P. CHIODO, MD
ERIC M. BLUMAN, MD, PhD

FOOT AND ANKLE CLINICS

www.foot.theclinics.com

Consulting Editor
MARK S. MYERSON, MD

September 2011 • Volume 16 • Number 3

SAUNDERS an imprint of ELSEVIER, Inc.

W.B. SAUNDERS COMPANY
A Division of Elsevier Inc.

1600 John F. Kennedy Blvd. • Suite 1800 • Philadelphia, PA 19103-2899

http://www.theclinics.com

FOOT AND ANKLE CLINICS Volume 16, Number 3
March 2011 ISSN 1083-7515, ISBN-13: 978-1-4557-0448-4

Editor: Yonah Korngold
Developmental Editor: Jessica Demetriou

Foot and Ankle Clinics (ISSN 1083-7515) is published quarterly by Elsevier, Inc., 360 Park Avenue South, New York, NY 10010-1710. Months of issue are March, June, September, and December. Periodicals postage paid at New York, NY, and additional mailing offices. Subscription price per year is $271.00 (US individuals), $357.00 (US institutions), $134.00 (US students), $308.00 (Canadian individuals), $422.00 (Canadian institutions), $184.00 (Canadian students), $397.00 (foreign individuals), $422.00 (foreign institutions), and $184.00 (foreign students). To receive student/resident rate, orders must be accompanied by name of affiliated institution, date of term, and the signature of program/residency coordinator on institution letterhead. Orders will be billed at individual rate until proof of status is received. Foreign air speed delivery is included in all *Clinics* subscription prices. All prices are subject to change without notice. **POSTMASTER:** Send address changes to *Foot and Ankle Clinics,* Elsevier Health Sciences Division, Subscription Customer Service, 3251 Riverport Lane, Maryland Heights, MO 63043. **Customer Service: 1-800-654-2452 (US and Canada). From outside of the United States and Canada, call 314-447-8871. Fax: 314-447-8029. E-mail: JournalsCustomerService-usa@elsevier.com (for print support); JournalsOnlineSupport-usa@elsevier.com (for online support).**

Reprints. For copies of 100 or more, of articles in this publication, please contact the Commercial Reprints Department, Elsevier Inc., 360 Park Avenue South, New York, NY 10010-1710. Tel.: 212-633-3812; Fax: 212-462-1935; E-mail: reprints@elsevier.com.

Printed and bound by CPI Group (UK) Ltd, Croydon, CR0 4YY

Transferred to Digital Print 2011

Contributors

CONSULTING EDITOR

MARK S. MYERSON, MD
Director, Institute for Foot and Ankle Reconstruction at Mercy, Mercy Medical Center, Baltimore, Maryland

GUEST EDITORS

CHRISTOPHER P. CHIODO, MD
Brigham Foot and Ankle Center, Department of Orthopaedics, Brigham and Women's Hospital, Boston, Massachusetts

ERIC M. BLUMAN, MD, PhD
Research Director, Brigham Foot and Ankle Center, Department of Orthopaedics, Brigham & Women's Hospital; Assistant Professor of Orthopaedics, Harvard Medical School, Boston, Massachusetts

AUTHORS

CHRISTOPHER BIBBO, DO, DPM, FACS, FAAOS, FACFAS
Chief, Foot & Ankle Section, Department of Orthopaedics, Marshfield Clinic, Marshfield, Wisconsin

ERIC M. BLUMAN, MD, PhD
Research Director, Brigham Foot and Ankle Center, Department of Orthopaedics, Brigham & Women's Hospital; Assistant Professor of Orthopaedics, Harvard Medical School, Boston, Massachusetts

MICHAEL A. CAMPBELL, MD
Foot and Ankle Fellow 2010–2011, Department of Orthopaedic Surgery, Penn State Milton S. Hershey Medical Center, Hershey Pennsylvania; Atlantic Orthopaedic Specialists, TRC Center, Virginia Beach, Virginia

BRIAN E. CLOWERS, MD
Institute for Foot and Ankle Reconstruction at Mercy, Mercy Medical Center, Baltimore, Maryland

THOMAS DOWD, MD
Brigham Foot and Ankle Center, Department of Orthopaedics, Brigham & Women's Hospital, Boston, Massachusetts

PAULO N. FERRAO, FCS(ortho) SA
Institute for Foot and Ankle Reconstruction at Mercy, Mercy Medical Center, Baltimore, Maryland

L. NATHAN GAUSE, MD
Campbell Clinic Foundation, University of Tennessee-Campbell Clinic, Memphis, Tennessee

SAMARJIT S. JAGLAN, MD, FAAOS
Chief, Pediatric Orthopaedic Section, Department of Orthopaedics, Marshfield Clinic, Marshfield, Wisconsin

PAUL J. JULIANO, MD
Professor of Orthopaedic Surgery; Head of Foot and Ankle Division; Residency and Foot and Ankle Fellowship Director, Penn State College of Medicine, Milton S. Hershey Medical Center, Hershey Pennsylvania

MARY ANN KEENAN, MD
Department of Orthopaedic Surgery, University of Pennsylvania School of Medicine, Philadelphia, Pennsylvania

STUART H. MYERS, MD
Resident, Department of Medicine, Johns Hopkins School of Medicine, Baltimore, Maryland

MARK S. MYERSON, MD
Director, Institute for Foot and Ankle Reconstruction at Mercy, Mercy Medical Center, Baltimore, Maryland

MICHAEL S. PINZUR, MD
Professor of Orthopaedic Surgery, Loyola University Health System, Maywood, Illinois

DAVID R. RICHARDSON, MD
Program Director, UT-Campbell Clinic Orthopaedic Surgery, Campbell Clinic Foundation, University of Tennessee-Campbell Clinic, Memphis, Tennessee

DANIEL B. RYSSMAN, MD
Department of Orthopedics, Mayo Clinic, Rochester, Minnesota

LEW C. SCHON, MD
Attending and Director, Foot and Ankle Service, Department of Orthopaedic Surgery, Union Memorial Hospital, Baltimore, Maryland

Contents

> This article serves as in introduction to the appreciation of the effects of motor imbalance on the foot during walking. A spectrum of disease ranging from paralysis to simple motor imbalance, to significant spastic motor imbalance, can be seen. A central goal is to create a stable platform to support weight bearing and/or locomotion. Several principles to achieve this are discussed. When bracing does not provide satisfactory results, tendon transfers may help. Concomitant procedures including motor unit lengthening, capsular releases, and osteotomies may also need to be performed.

> Tendon transfers are powerful procedures that have demonstrated the ability to restore substantial function to appropriately selected patients. However, there are important procedural considerations and inherent limitations to acknowledge before the use of these techniques. Tendon transfers are optimally performed within a healthy soft tissue bed, across mobile joints, and using proper donor tissue. Appropriate tensioning and insertion points must be chosen. Finally, perioperative care should include appropriate immobilization, subsequent rehabilitation, analgesics, and avoidance of nicotine. A thorough understanding and proper implementation of these concepts will optimize outcomes.

> Equinovarus deformity results in a foot and ankle posture that makes it nearly impossible to ambulate correctly, stand at ease, or even allow appropriate orthotic/prosthetic. Tendon transfer surgery remains a mainstay to treat equinovarus deformity, resulting in improved balance, posture and gait. This chapter describes the etiologies, evaluation and operative management of equinovarus deformity in adult and pediatric populations.

The "bridle" procedure is a modification of the transfer of the tibialis posterior to the dorsum of the foot for the treatment of a supple equinus or equinovarus deformity of the ankle and hindfoot. Indications vary based on the underlying pathology, but is indicated primarily in the setting of a drop-foot and a steppage gait, which is awkward, energy consuming, and physically limiting. This procedure usually allows for brace-free ambulation while minimizing the risk of recurrent deformity. However, the patient and family must understand a "normal" gait is unusual.

Correction of the adult cavovarus foot deformity, whether rigid or flexible, can be quite challenging. While there are many causes of this deformity, the universal problem is the loss of muscle balance. If untreated, progression of deformity is inevitable, and generally the flexible deformity becomes rigid. It makes sense to commence treatment as early as possible, but this is not always realistic. When surgery is indicated, the goal is to obtain a plantigrade *and* balanced foot, which cannot be accomplished without tendon transfers. The foot and ankle must be in equilibrium, and tendon transfers are an integral addition for correction.

Deformities of the hallux can be quite disabling; malalignment can lead to both pain and dysfunction. Tendon transfers have become an invaluable tool in the treatment of several hallux deformities. This article addresses the use of tendon transfer for 2 common deformities, hallux varus and clawing of the hallux.

Lesser toe deformities can be successfully corrected surgically. Forefoot tendon transfers are more technically demanding, but are uniquely able to provide dynamic stability to the lesser toes after correction. We describe our technique for 2 such procedures: flexor transfer and extensor digitorum brevis (EDB) transfer. In addition to discussion of the technical aspects of these procedures, we address the historical perspective, indications, contraindications, preoperative planning, complications, postoperative management, results, as well as our concerns regarding the technique and its future.

> The correction of the paralytic equinovalgus deformity is a challenging problem that, when preformed well, can be very satisfying for both surgeon and the patient. Treatment goals are to create a stable, plantigrade, and functional foot that does not require bracing. It is important to adhere to the basic principles of tendon transfer. Make the patient aware that intensive muscle retraining is required in the rehabilitation phase. With careful preoperative planning, appropriate bony procedures, and functional tendon transfers, good results are achievable.

> Spastic equinovarus foot deformity is common in patients with upper motor neuron syndrome following stroke and traumatic brain injury. Equinovarus posture of the foot causes significant problems with shoe wear, standing, transfers, and walking. The deformity often cannot be managed with nonsurgical treatments such as chemodenervation, orthoses, and physical therapy. In fact, these modalities may be more costly and less effective than surgical treatment This article describes evaluation and surgical techniques of combined multitendon transfers and lengthenings for correction of spastic equinovarus deformity. These tendon transfers reliably result in improvement in quality of life.

THE CLINICS ARE NOW AVAILABLE ONLINE!

Access your subscription at:
www.theclinics.com

Foreword

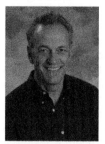

Mark S. Myerson, MD
Consulting Editor

The uses of tendon transfers is a fascinating topic. Although we do not treat as many paralytic deformities as were corrected surgically in the era of polio, there are many circumstances where tendon transfers remain an essential part of the operative management of deformity. The correction of foot and ankle deformity by means of a correctly performed tendon transfer can be satisfying for both the surgeon and the patient. The goal of any tendon transfer is to create a stable, functioning, and plantigrade foot, and this goal applies to every tendon transfer performed for paralysis because the correction of deformity, the improvement of function, and the establishment of a plantigrade foot are essential.

I would like to consider the patient with cavoequinovarus deformity, the result of hereditary sensory motor neuropathy (CMT), as an illustrative example of mismanagement of deformity correction. I have learned over the decades that a triple arthrodesis is an excellent procedure, provided the foot is correctly balanced with additional osteotomy and tendon transfer. The triple arthrodesis gained a poor reputation for correction of the cavus foot since recurrent deformity was common. However, for the majority of these patients for whom deformity recurred, no tendon transfer was performed because it was felt that the posterior tendon tibial tendon for example was too weak to be of any benefit. However, the posterior tibial tendon inserts distal to the talonavicular joint, and unless the tendon is transferred, the medial foot deformity will gradually recur into adductovarus or equinovarus. Integral to the success of any of these procedures is a corrected foot, a plantigrade hindfoot relative to the forefoot, and muscle balance. Even with perfectly executed surgery, if the posterior tibial muscle is overactive relative to the evertors of the hindfoot, the foot will ultimately deform. Even though the posterior tibial muscle may not be strong enough to support a paralytic equinus deformity, it should nonetheless be transferred, usually to the dorsum of the foot.

When any tendon transfer is planned, one must consider the relative muscle strengths and tendon excursion of every functioning muscle, no matter how weak it may appear; the positioning of the tendon to be transferred relative to the rest of the foot; the proper tensioning of a transferred tendon; and the pull-out strength necessary to secure the tendon transfer. Optimally, a tendon transfer should

Foot Ankle Clin N Am 16 (2011) ix–xi
doi:10.1016/j.fcl.2011.06.007
1083-7515/11/$ – see front matter © 2011 Elsevier Inc. All rights reserved.

approximate the strength and excursion of the motor unit it is trying to replace, but this can be rarely accomplished with a single tendon. Therefore expecting the extensor hallucis longus muscle to replace the anterior tibial muscle, or the flexor digitorum longus muscle to replace the posterior tibial muscle, is unrealistic.

Most muscles will lose a grade of power when transferred, particularly if the transfer is not phasic (a tendon that is primarily a flexor and is transferred to function as an extensor). As an example, a PTT transfer to the dorsum of the foot to regain dorsiflexion strength is not phasic, and muscle power is lost. It is always preferable to use a muscle that is phasic because less "reeducation" of the muscle is required, rehabilitation is facilitated, and less strength of the muscle is lost in the transfer. Typically in a PTT transfer performed through the interosseous membrane to the dorsum of the foot for correction of a flaccid paralysis muscle strength is lost. The same applies to another nonphasic transfer such as the peroneal muscle(s) to substitute for absent ankle dorsiflexion. I have been very encouraged with the use of nonstandard tendon transfers. Basically, if there is deformity as a result of tendon imbalance, transfer the involved tendon, even if it is slightly weak. Where you transfer it to is not as important as removing the deforming force. A tendon transfer will then have two benefits: the one is the removal of the deforming force and thereby lessening deformity, and the second is to take advantage of the muscle that is transferred to further improve the function of the foot. A good example of this is the transfer of the flexor hallucis longus (FHL) to the base of the proximal phalanx for correction of a flexible claw hallux deformity. By removing the FHL from its attachment to the distal phalanx, the flexion effect on the interphalangeal joint is minimized, and the transfer into the base of the proximal phalanx increases flexion strength of the hallux since the intrinsic muscles (in this case, the flexor hallucis brevis) are rarely functioning.

It is difficult to know how tight the tendon transfer is to be when secured to the bone. If it is fixed at maximal elongation, the tendon transfer acts more like a tenodesis, although it always stretches out. However, if it is fixed in its relaxed state, it cannot generate adequate tension to pull effectively. Generally, I prefer to insert the tendon under more tension than relaxation because some stretching out of the muscle always occurs. The converse however does not apply, and muscle strength can never be regained if the transfer is too loose. Finally, if transferred underneath a retinaculum that functions as a pulley, this increases the effective tendon excursion (range of motion). However, this transfer brings the tendon closer to the ankle or subtalar axes and diminishes the lever arm and the subsequent strength of the transfer. With a subcutaneous position of a tendon transfer, excursion is decreased, but motor strength is maximized because of the greater distance from the joint axes and the resulting greater lever arm. In general, a tendon is always transferred in a subcutaneous position. Quite apart from the biomechanical advantage outlined here, there is a greater likelihood of the tendon ultimately getting stuck if the transfer is performed under the retinaculum.

Wherever possible, I perform a transfer using a tunnel with a bone tendon–bone interference fit of the tendon. A more simple attachment of the tendon to the periosteum is never as secure. This does mean however that sufficient tendon length is present in order to insert the tendon in the correct location, but simultaneously has enough length to insert it into a bone tunnel. The options for securing the tendon in the tunnel include an interference fit with a bone peg, a screw, either metallic or bioresorbable, or a suture anchor. Generally, I use both since most of these patients have relative osteopenia and I do not think that an interference screw provides adequate fixation to support the transfer. This fixation of the tendon is very important, since rehabilitation with weight-bearing and passive range-of-motion exercises may begin once the sutures are removed, and the strengthening and reeducation that needs to be initiated may start sooner. Rehabilitation is essential regardless of the type of transfer, although this is easier to accomplish if the transferred tendon is in phase with the muscle it replaced.

Mark S. Myerson, MD
Institute for Foot and Ankle Reconstruction at Mercy
Mercy Medical Center
301 St. Paul Place
Baltimore, MD 21202, USA

E-mail address:
mark4feet@aol.com

Preface

Tendon transfers have been an invaluable part of the orthopedic armamentarium for more than a century. These procedures have great utility in correcting deformity, establishing or augmenting motor function, and generating a tenodesis effect. As such, they have become some of the most frequently performed orthopedic foot and ankle surgeries. Their success provides great satisfaction to both patient and surgeon alike.

Despite their utility and longevity, there remains a relative paucity of literature on many aspects of tendon transfers about the foot and ankle. Perhaps this is because there is just as much art as science to performing tendon transfers, or maybe it is due to the degree of difficulty in performing properly balanced procedures. Certainly, there are few, if any, cookbook approaches to a successful tendon transfer.

Fortunately, foot and ankle orthopedic surgery is replete with the wisdom and knowledge of many individuals with vast personal experience in this area. We are honored to have several leading clinicians in the field of tendon transfers about the foot and ankle as contributors to this issue. We thank them profoundly for the time and effort they put forth to complete this issue. Their expertise not only will provide useful clinical insight but also hopefully will spur further research and clinical advances in this rewarding field.

Christopher P. Chiodo, MD
Eric M. Bluman, MD, PhD

Brigham Foot and Ankle Center
Department of Orthopaedics
Brigham and Women's Hospital
75 Francis Street
Boston, MA 02115, USA

E-mail addresses:
cchiodo@partners.org
ebluman@partners.org

Foot Ankle Clin N Am 16 (2011) xiii
doi:10.1016/j.fcl.2011.08.002
1083-7515/11/$ – see front matter © 2011 Elsevier Inc. All rights reserved.

Principles of Balancing the Foot with Tendon Transfers

Michael S. Pinzur, MD

KEYWORDS
• Balance • Tendon transfer • Walking • Weight bearing

The foot is the unique end organ of weight bearing that functions as an essential component of normal efficient walking. It has an adaptable bony architecture that allows prepositioning of its durable plantar soft tissue envelope in a plantigrade position to accept the impact of loading. It is then capable of transitioning during stance phase from the pressure-dissipating unlocked position at heel strike to the locked position at push-off that optimizes stable propulsion. Underactivity or overactivity of the motors that drive this process leads to inefficiency and/or instability during walking.

MOTOR TESTING

Most of our understanding of the foot without motor balance was developed during the era of poliomyelitis. The first step in planning a tendon transfer is identification of the motors available both in the direction of correction (agonist) and the direction of deformity (antagonist). It is a good practice to create a worksheet with a list of deficits on one side of the page and available motors on the opposite side. Muscles are graded as shown in **Table 1**.

ACHIEVING MOTOR BALANCE ACROSS A JOINT

There are several basic principles that must be respected when approaching the motor unbalanced joint. First, joint excursion can only be accomplished within the realm of the available passive motion present. Tendon transfer cannot correct a static deformity, that is, a fixed joint contracture. Soft tissue release or corrective osteotomy must be achieved before or at the time of tendon transfer surgery. Second, tendon transfers generally perform optimally when the transferred motor unit normally functions during the same functional phase of activity as the deficient motor. When an "in-phase" motor is not available, then the best "out-of-phase" motor is the next best option.

Third, motor unit transfer often looses 1 grade of muscle strength after surgical transfer, so tendon transfer is rarely entertained when the transferred muscle is less

Department of Orthopaedic Surgery, Loyola University Health Center, 2160 South First Avenue, Maywood, IL 60153, USA
E-mail address: mpinzu1@lumc.edu

Foot Ankle Clin N Am 16 (2011) 375–384
doi:10.1016/j.fcl.2011.06.001
1083-7515/11/$ – see front matter © 2011 Elsevier Inc. All rights reserved.

Table 1
Muscle grading

Numeric Grade	Descriptive Grade	Description
0	None	No muscle contraction.
1	Trace	Contraction is palpable and may be visible, but there is no active motion of the affected joint.
2	Poor	The muscle is actively able to move the affected joint, but is not capable of achieving motion against gravity.
3	Fair	The muscle is able to move the joint through its full range and against gravity, but not against resistance.
4	Good	The muscle is capable of moving the joint through a full range and against some, but not normal, resistance.
5	Normal	The muscle is capable of moving the joint through a full range against normal resistance.

than grade 4. Transferred tendons should be anchored under tension, to maximize mechanical efficiency. When a transferred tendon is split and attached to 2 insertion points, the slip under the greater tension functions far more efficiently. Fourth, transferred muscles should course in a straight direction and be routed through subcutaneous tissue. When a transferred muscle is required to be routed about a pulley, it is either weakened by the turn, or tethers and eventually ruptures from the involved friction. A subcutaneous passage allows the tendon to glide. A tendon that is transferred over exposed bleeding bone is likely to become tethered owing to adhesions, limiting tendon excursion and transfer function. Finally, there should be sufficient excursion of the transferred tendon to move the target joint through a functional range of motion.

CREATING A STABLE PLATFORM TO SUPPORT WEIGHT BEARING

A unique requirement of the unbalanced foot is the necessity for achieving a plantigrade foot by the end of treatment. This may require osteotomy, arthrodesis, soft tissue release, or a combination of these. This principle cannot be overemphasized and failure to do so can jeopardize the outcome.

PARALYSIS

The most common paralytic foot problem that currently presents to the orthopaedic surgeon is traumatic peroneal palsy, more commonly described as foot drop. This condition arises from traumatic injury to the peroneal nerve, leaving the individual with paralysis of the muscles in the anterior and lateral compartments of the leg. Patients seek medical attention for this disorder owing to tripping over a plantarflexed foot during swing phase of gait. Initial treatment should be with an ankle foot orthosis (AFO) that blocks ankle plantarflexion. An AFO can be fabricated from modern plastics or with the classic double upright construction. When used long term, either form can be enhanced with dorsiflexion assist and plantarflexion stop parameters (**Fig. 1**).

Surgery may be performed to resolve static equinus contracture of the ankle joint, or when the patient desires to walk without a brace. Patients occasionally develop static ankle equinus owing to contracture of the gastrocnemius-soleus motor unit or

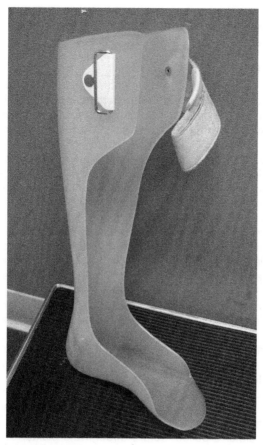

Fig. 1. Standard polypropylene AFO.

the posterior ankle joint capsule. Depending on the source of the deformity, conventional treatment for static ankle equinus is musculotendinous lengthening of the gastrocnemius-soleus muscle unit, percutaneous lengthening of the Achilles tendon, or posterior ankle capsular release. Proponents of circular fine-wire fixation have advocated the use of gradual correction with a dynamic fixator. Once corrected, treatment with an orthosis can be reinstituted.

Tendon transfer surgery can be entertained for patients who find treatment with an orthosis to be suboptimal. Patients considering tendon transfer surgery should be informed that the goal of surgery is to achieve function that approaches walking with the AFO. The functional motor deficit in foot-drop is from paralysis of the tibialis anterior, which is the primary ankle dorsiflexor. Because motor strength and power are directly correlated with cross-sectional area, the best available motor unit to treat paralytic foot-drop is the tibialis posterior. Several methods of transferring the posterior tibial tendon to the dorsum of the foot have been described. The most efficient method of achieving active dorsiflexion power is transfer of the posterior tibial tendon through the interosseous membrane to the dorsum of the foot.[1] The tendon is then secured to the midfoot through a drill hole distal to the dorsiflexion axis. A second method, the "bridle procedure," attaches the posterior tibial tendon to the anterior tibial tendon.[2] The bridle procedure is often performed in conjunction with subcutaneous transfer of 1 or both peroneal tendons superficial to the distal fibula.

Operative Techniques

The first step with either method requires correction of the static ankle equinus contracture. This can be achieved by either percutaneous triple hemisection of the Achilles tendon (Hoke procedure), or fractional muscle lengthening of the gastrocnemius, (Strayer procedure). The tendon of the tibialis posterior muscle is sharply detached from its insertion on the tubercle of the navicular and the spring ligament, taking care to preserve as much length as possible. A second incision is then made overlying the musculotendinous junction of the tibialis posterior along the posteromedial border of the tibia. A superficial posterior compartment fasciotomy is performed. The distal tendon is freed from all attachments in the distal wound and then retracted into the proximal posterior wound. An incision is then made overlying the anterior compartment in line with the direction of the transferred tendon, followed by an anterior compartment fasciotomy. A curved, 6-inch hemostat is then passed along the posterior border of the tibia, where it is used to penetrate the interosseous membrane and create a defect to pass the tendon transfer. Heavy suture is placed through the tibialis posterior tendon before transfer through the interosseous membrane into the anterior compartment incision. An incision is then made overlying the "neutral dorsiflexion point" in the foot, where the tendon is attached. This location is determined by gentle pressure on the plantar surface of the foot in line with the direction of pull for the transferred tibialis posterior. A drill hole can be made at this point, which is generally within the middle cuneiform. This location is occasionally though 1 of the joints of the middle cuneiform. The hole is enlarged to accept the transferred tendon. A large hemostat is then used to create a straight subcutaneous tunnel for passing the tendon from the anterior incision to the dorsal foot incision. The tendon can then be attached with either a pullout suture through the plantar surface of the foot (where it is tied over a felt bolster), or with an interference screw (**Fig. 2**). The paralyzed anterior tendon can also be transferred for 2 possible reasons: (1) To provide substance for securing the tibialis posterior tendon, which is generally barely of sufficient length to enter the drill hole, and/or (2) to act as a static tenodesis to resist passive plantar flexion during the period of time when the tibialis posterior will need to "learn" to become a swing phase dorsiflexor.[1] The alternative "bridle" method attaches the tibialis posterior to the anteriorly transferred peroneal muscles, which are all secured to the tibialis anterior tendon.[2] This is discussed elsewhere in this issue.

A splint is applied in the operating room, immobilizing the ankle in neutral or slight dorsiflexion. A short leg walking cast can be applied at the first clinic visit, taking care to pad the dorsal region of the foot and ankle where the transferred tendons are superficial and prone to pressure ulcers. If an anchoring suture is used, it is removed at 6 to 8 weeks after surgery, when the patient is transitioned to an AFO for 6 to 12 months. This is necessary to accommodate the 9- to 12-month "learning period" during which the transferred tibialis posterior muscle "learns" to become a swing phase dorsiflexor.[1]

MOTOR IMBALANCE

Isolated dynamic varus or valgus occurs owing to a dynamic motor imbalance between the hindfoot invertors (posterior tibialis, tibialis anterior) and evertors

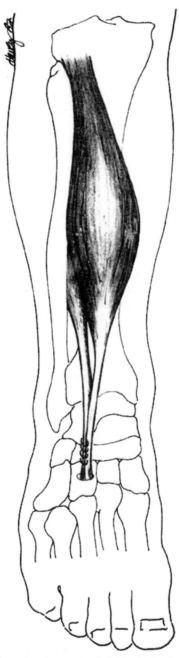

Fig. 2. The posterior tibial tendon is rerouted through the interosseous membrane and attached to a drill hole at the "neutral dorsiflexion point" in the foot. The anterior tibial tendon can also be transferred to act as a tenodesis during the healing period, and to augment fixation of the posterior tibial tendon which barely has sufficient length to enter the drill hole. (*From* Pinzur MS, Kett N, Trilla M. Combined anterior/posterior tibial tendon transfer in post-traumatic peroneal palsy. Foot Ankle 1988;8:273; with permission.)

(peroneal muscles). Again, the first step is to determine whether a static or dynamic equinus force is present, and whether active dorsiflexion is present. When the patient has no dynamic dorsiflexion, the 2 options are soft tissue release and bracing (with an AFO) or tendon transfer as described. Gastrocnemius or Achilles tendon lengthening is the first step when the gastrocnemius-soleus muscle group overpowers the foot and ankle dorsiflexors.

There are 2 surgical options when an AFO is not capable of controlling the instability, or when the patient would like to avoid using an AFO. The first option is a fractional muscle lengthening of the deforming muscle or muscle group to create motor balance. This may be accomplished by fractional muscle lengthening of the tibialis anterior in dynamic varus or peroneal muscles in dynamic valgus. A short-leg walking cast is used postoperatively to allow the lengthened motor units to "find" their correct length. Patients can be gradually transitioned to an AFO.

Occasionally, the dynamic varus or valgus is from antagonist motor group paralysis. In this situation, the deforming muscle is best transferred to the "neutral dorsiflexion point" to avoid late recurrence of the deformity.

SPASTICITY

A combination of static and dynamic deformity can be created by brain injury owing to stroke (cerebral vascular accident) or closed brain injury. Surgery is avoided early in the recovery phase of either disorder, utilizing standard physical therapy programs and appropriate AFO bracing techniques. Intervention is delayed until patients either plateau in their recovery or deformity impedes their rehabilitation.

The most typical deformity in adults is adult-acquired spastic equinovarus. This deformity can be thought of as decorticate posturing during walking. The gait abnormality is primarily due to the spastic equinus during stance phase. The spastic equinus produces a toe–heel gait pattern as opposed to the normal heel–toe pattern. Hyperextension later occurs at the knee joint to accommodate the spastic ankle equinus during mid and terminal stance phase of gait. Children with cerebral palsy accommodate this spastic deformity by walking on their toes. Adults do not possess adequate balance to "toe-walk," so they develop a hyperextension "back-knee" deformity with increasing spastic ankle joint equinus. When the spastic ankle joint equinus reaches a critical magnitude, patients are not able to advance their contralateral normal limb past the involved limb during swing phase (**Fig. 3**).[3,4]

The first step in treatment of adult-acquired spastic equinovarus is physical therapy gait training and a rigid AFO. When the orthosis is not capable of controlling the deformity, motor balancing surgery is a reasonable option. Surgery should not be offered until the patient has reached a plateau with standard rehabilitation techniques. This period until recovery is approximately 6 months after cerebral vascular accident and 12 to 18 months after closed brain injury.

Operative Technique

The first step in achieving muscle balance is achieved with either fractional muscle lengthening of the gastrocnemius-soleus muscle group or percutaneous triple hemisection of the Achilles tendon (**Fig. 4**). The varus component is addressed by either lateral transfer of the tibialis anterior to the "neutral dorsiflexion point," or split anterior tibial tendon transfer.

Lateral transfer of the tibialis anterior tendon is accomplished through 3 small incisions. The tendon is detached from its insertion on the dorsomedial foot. A

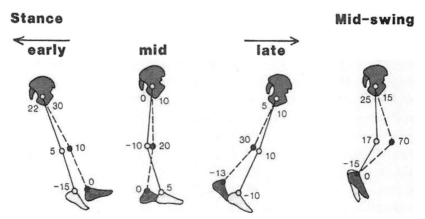

Fig. 3. Composite electrogoniometric data of a composite group of hemiplegic patients (*solid*) compared with our laboratory control population (*dash*), at 4 times in the gait cycle. Note that the primary deformity is ankle equinus (plantar flexion) at initial floor contact (heel strike). (*From* Pinzur MS, Sherman R, DiMonte-Levine P, et al. Gait Changes in adult onset hemiplegia. Am J Phys Med 1987;66:235; with permission.)

small incision is made over the musculotendinous junction of the tibialis anterior, where the tendon is retracted. The tendon is then rerouted subcutaneously where it is attached to the "neutral dorsiflexion point" with either a pull-out suture or an interference screw (**Fig. 5**). Severe stance-phase varus can also be improved by additionally performing a fractional muscle lengthening of the tibialis posterior, flexor hallucis longus, and flexor digitorum longus motor units. Postoperative

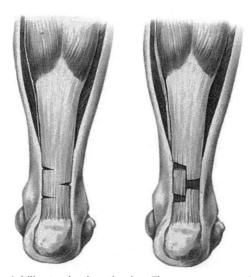

Fig. 4. Percutaneous Achilles tendon lengthening. Three percutaneous hemi-transections of the Achilles tendon are performed through 2 medial and one lateral stab wound with a #11 scalpel blade. (*From* Pinzur MS. In: Kelikian AS, editor. Amputations of the foot and ankle. Stamford (CT): Appleton & Lange; 1999. p. 615; with permission.)

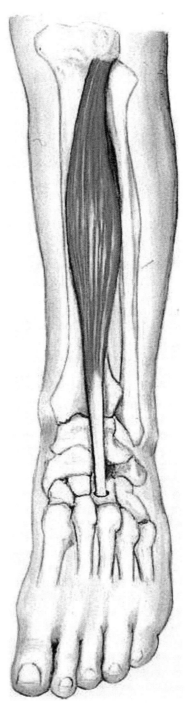

Fig. 5. Lateral transfer of the tibialis anterior for adult acquired spastic equinovarus. (*From* Pinzur MS, Sherman R, DiMonte-Levine P, et al. Adult-onset hemiplegia, gait changes after muscle-balancing procedures to correct the equinus. J Bone Joint Surg 1986;68A:1254; with permission.)

HEMIPLEGIC LIMB POST–OP
vs. CONTROL POPULATION

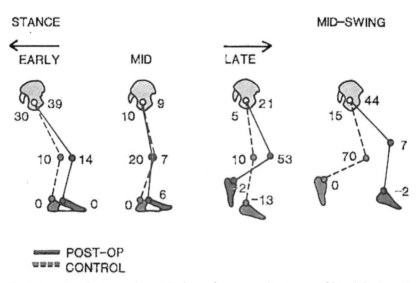

STANCE   MID–SWING

← EARLY   MID   LATE →

━━━ POST–OP
▬▬▬ CONTROL

Fig. 6. Composite electrogoniometric data of a composite group of hemiplegic patients after surgical correction of adult acquired spastic equinovarus (*solid*) compared with our laboratory control population (*dash*), at a minimum of 1 year after surgery. (*From* Pinzur MS, Sherman R, DiMonte-Levine P, et al. Adult-onset hemiplegia, gait changes after muscle-balancing procedures to correct the equinus. J Bone Joint Surg 1986;68A:1256; with permission.)

management is similar to the treatment after posterior tibial tendon transfer for traumatic peroneal palsy.[3]

The split anterior tibial tendon transfer procedure is performed by transferring one third to one half of the tibialis anterior tendon, and attaching it to the cuboid. This creates a dorsiflexion sling.[5]

Although gait does not return to normal after this surgery, the knee hyperextension moment is generally eliminated, and walking stability is greatly improved **(Fig. 6)**.[3,5]

DISCUSSION

This article serves as in introduction to the appreciation of the effects of motor imbalance on the foot during walking. A spectrum of disease ranging from paralysis to simple motor imbalance, to significant spastic motor imbalance, can be seen. A central goal is to create a stable platform to support weight bearing and/or locomotion. Several principles to achieve this are discussed. When bracing does not provide satisfactory results, tendon transfers may help. Concomitant procedures including motor unit lengthening, capsular releases, and osteotomies may also need to be performed.

REFERENCES

1. Pinzur MS, Kett N, Trilla M. Combined anterior/posterior tibial tendon transfer in post-traumatic peroneal palsy. Foot Ankle 1988;8:271–5.
2. Rodriguez RP. The bridle procedure in the treatment of paralysis of the foot. Foot Ankle 1992;13:63–9.
3. Pinzur MS, Sherman R, DiMonte Levine P, et al. Adult onset hemiplegia, gait changes after muscle balancing procedures to correct the equinus. J Bone Joint Surg 1986; 68A:1249–57.
4. Pinzur MS, Sherman R, DiMonte-Levine P, et al. Gait changes in adult onset hemiplegia. Am J Phys Med 1987;66:228–37.
5. Keenan MA, Creighton J, Garland DE, et al. Surgical correction of spastic equinovarus deformity in the adult head trauma patient. Foot Ankle 1984;5:35–41.

The Basics and Science of Tendon Transfers

Eric M. Bluman, MD, PhD*, Thomas Dowd, MD

KEYWORDS
- Tendon suspension • Interface • Balance • Fixation
- Tension • Transplantation

Tendon transfers are an invaluable tool that may be used for a variety of purposes in foot and ankle surgery. They allow for the correction of deformity, establishment or augmentation of motor function, or the generation of a tenodesis effect. These procedures are especially effective for correcting supple deformities caused by dynamic muscular imbalance.[1]

HISTORY

Tendon transfer procedures have been utilized in orthopaedics for at least 130 years. The first described transfer was of the peroneus longus muscle by Nicoladoni in 1882.[2] Although this procedure failed, a high level of interest in Europe was generated by Nicoladoni's stature as the chairman of the Department of Surgery at the University of Innsbruck as well as the overwhelming need to combat the effects of poliomyelitis. By the end of the 19th century, a number of others had started to contribute to the field.[3,4] At the time, many of the indications for these procedures were improper, muscles transferred were inadequate, and the techniques suboptimal. Although a number of individuals made early contributions, it was Mayer[5] who described many of the principles of tendon transfers still in use today. Mayer's 5 main principles were:

1. Restore the normal relationship between tendon and sheath.
2. Have the tendon course through tissue that is adapted to gliding of the tendon.
3. Imitate normal insertion of the tendon.
4. Establish normal tension.
5. Create an effective line of traction.

Since this early work, a multitude of tendon transfer procedures have been described in many orthopaedic subspecialties. Despite a rich history of over a century of clinical use and the current ubiquity of these procedures in many orthopaedic subspecialties, there is a lack of basic science to guide us toward best practice in their execution.

Brigham Foot and Ankle Center, Department of Orthopaedics, Brigham & Women's Hospital, 75 Francis Street, Boston, MA 02115, USA
* Corresponding author.
E-mail address: ebluman@partners.org

Foot Ankle Clin N Am 16 (2011) 385–399
doi:10.1016/j.fcl.2011.06.002
1083-7515/11/$ – see front matter © 2011 Elsevier Inc. All rights reserved.

foot.theclinics.com

This article incorporates literature from all orthopaedic subspecialties in an effort to glean useful data that may be applied to tendon transfers about the foot and ankle.

NOMENCLATURE

There have been a number of terms used to describe the procedures by which motor units are surgically modified to improve function. It is important to delineate the terms and their definitions to avoid confusion.

A *tendon transfer* is the detachment of the tendon of a functioning muscle at its insertion with subsequent relocation to a new insertion or attachment. Tendon transfers about the foot and ankle often involve the movement of a functional, deforming tendon to a position of greater utility.[6] Most of the topics covered in this issue fall under this category.

A *tendon translocation* describes the rerouting of a tendon, without detachment of the origin or insertion, to modify its function. Although classically referred to as a tenosuspension, Young's procedure is an example of a tendon translocation. This procedure is employed in the treatment of adult-acquired flatfoot deformity, whereby the anterior tibialis tendon is rerouted plantarly through a slot created in the navicular.[7] Another example is Makin's translocation of the flexor pollicis longus tendon dorsally and radially in the thumb to restore opposition.[8]

Muscle-tendon transplantation is performed when both the origin and insertion of the motor unit is detached with the accompanying neurovascular supply and implanted in a new location. An example of this is the transplantation of both the rectus femoris and vascularized iliac crest to restore ankle dorsiflexion and reconstruct a segmental tibial defect.[9] Additional examples include gracilis or contralateral latissimus dorsi free-functioning transplants for brachial plexus injury.[10]

Tendon suspension or *tenosuspension* procedures involve the use of a tendon to create support for a structure, such as the passage of a harvested peroneus longus tendon through the acromion and proximal humerus to stabilize the shoulder.[11] Examples in the lower extremity include the Jones and Hibbs tenosuspensions.[12]

EPIDEMIOLOGY

A number of orthopaedic subspecialties rely heavily on tendon transfers for optimization of outcomes. Hand surgery, orthopaedic foot and ankle surgery, and pediatric orthopaedics utilize these techniques most frequently. Surgeries for cerebral palsy, chronic Achilles tendon ruptures, and reconstruction of adult-acquired flat foot deformities among others regularly incorporate tendon transfers. As a result, tens of thousands of tendon transfer procedures are performed annually in the United States.

PLANNING AND PERFORMING TENDON TRANSFERS

The performance of tendon transfers should never be undertaken using a cookbook approach. However, there are guidelines by which to plan and perform these procedures. We first review the prerequisites to be fulfilled before undertaking the actual tendon transfer (**Box 1**). Once the prerequisites have been met, there are 5 basic principles that the surgeon should use to decide on the best motor to transfer for balance between the transfer and its opposing muscles (**Box 2**). Other factors are important to consider, even when the prerequisites and basic principles have been fulfilled are also discussed.

> **Box 1**
> **Prerequisites needed for successful tendon transfer**
>
> Analysis of the patient's needs and goals.
>
> Knowledge of the patient's appreciation of surgical expectations and limitations.
>
> Adequate soft tissue bed for coverage.
>
> Mobile intercalary joints.
>
> Donor motor unit that has adequate strength, sufficient excursion, and expendability.

Prerequisites for Successful Tendon Transfer

Analysis of the patient's needs and goals

With any orthopaedic treatment, the goals of the intervention should match the needs of the patient. Consider, for example, the use of a tendon transfer to improve ankle dorsiflexion in a wheelchair-bound patient with a painless flaccid paralysis who is effectively managed with an ankle–foot orthosis. This represents a procedure that is wasteful and places the patient at needless risk. Further, the realistic improvement that is expected needs to be understood by the patient before the surgery. It is important not to only go over what the patient can expect to gain, but also the limitations with which they will be left. This should be communicated multiple times before the surgery.

Adequate soft tissue bed for coverage

Transfers performed without adequate coverage will become desiccated, infected, or both. Adequate coverage is paramount when dealing with tendon transfers about the foot and ankle because many locations have a limited soft tissue envelope. Tenodeses, especially those involving weaves, take up more volume than the native local tissues and may lead to incision closure problems. Similarly, the quality of the soft tissue coverage must also be evaluated. A tendon transfer that can only be routed through soft tissue envelope that is heavily scarred is contraindicated.

Mobile intercalary joints

Without mobile joints the purposes of tendon transfers—correction of deformity, improvement of motor function, and creation of a tenodesis effect—cannot be accomplished and therefore should not be performed.

Bony and joint stability

Just as functional tendon transfers require mobile joints to effect their intended function, they also require bony and joint stability. Tendon transfers that span

> **Box 2**
> **Five basic principles to base decision on the best motor to transfer**
>
> Appropriate strength
>
> Appropriate amplitude
>
> Direction and attachment
>
> Integrity
>
> Synergy

unstable nonunions or pseudarthroses will fail or have less than their desired function. Similarly, some modicum of joint stability is required for success. A transfer acting on a joint without any stability will not have its desired effect. Even tendon transfers performed to increase joint stability require some degree of stability to act upon.

Donor motor unit qualities

A number of different criteria need to be fulfilled. The motor that is to be transferred needs to have adequate strength to perform the function that will be required. It is generally agreed that motor units lose at least one grade of muscle strength when transferred. Transferring muscles that already have compromised strength may limit their ability to function dynamically and result in their function being more of a tenodesis. Excursion also needs to be adequate. Generally, the problem encountered is lack of appropriate excursion. Such transfers may limit function because they will decrease motion and may eventually lead to joint contractures. This may eventually lead to joint contractures because of decreased motion. The motor transferred should also be expendable. The donor site from which the tendon is transferred will lose strength, function, or both. Essential functions should not be sacrificed. Any gain of function has to outweigh any loss that is incurred in the transfer. In some cases, it is appropriate to transfer an antagonist muscle, thereby not only adding strength to the desired function, but also weakening the antagonist function.

Basic Principles for Successful Tendon Transfer

Appropriate strength

There are 2 characteristics evaluated when determining whether the motor to be transferred will have appropriate strength. The amount of force that a muscle is capable of generating is proportional to its cross sectional area. The amount of force able to be generated is approximated by 3.6 kg/cm^2 or 50 lb/in^2. The motor unit to be transferred must have enough strength to perform the desired activity with a resting tone below that which would have it function as a tenodesis.

The work able to be performed is also important. Work that a muscle is able to generate is equal to the force it can generate multiplied by length of contraction. This is proportional to the product of the cross-sectional area and the fiber length. In essence, the capacity for work is related to the mass of the muscle transferred.

Appropriate amplitude

The amplitude of a musculotendinous unit is the magnitude of excursion that is able to be generated by muscular contraction. The *absolute amplitude* is the linear excursion observed when unaffected (ie, without the tendon passing through pulleys or over intercalary joints). The *effective amplitude* is the excursion of the musculotendinous unit as it is affected by the anatomy along its path. These anatomic modifiers change the resting length of the unit as well as the tension able to be generated and therefore modify the amplitude observed.

Direction and attachment

Tendon transfers should be in a straight line or as close to straight as possible. Careful consideration should go into a decision regarding the best insertion site. Insertion near the axis of rotation provides greater excursion but a diminished moment. Tendons transferred more distal on the lever arm reduce the excursion obtained, but produce a greater moment. In most cases, the superficial soft tissue envelope and the need to prevent bowstringing of the tendon limit how far one may set the distal attachment. Pulleys, although infrequently used in foot and ankle surgery, should be stable and straight.

Synergy and phase of muscle transfer

Tendon transfers may be placed to act "in-phase" or "out-of-phase." Most orthopaedic surgeons have heard this terminology, but many have a hard time explaining exactly what it means. The terminology derives from the gait cycle. The two main phases of the gait cycle are swing and stance. In each of these phases, there are characteristic muscle groups that undergo contraction while others are at rest. Simply stated, a tendon transfer is considered in-phase if it its muscle contracts during the expected motion. A muscle is out of phase if it is at rest during an expected motion or is activated at another stage of the motion.[13]

Optimization of tendon transfer requires the transferred tendon to act in-phase. In-phase muscle transfers fire with their native group to produce the desired effect, training or reeducation is minimal if needed at all. Out-of-phase transfers are not contraindicated; they are just not optimal. For proper functioning the out-of-phase muscle transfer must undergo reeducation, which may be slow and can take several months.[1]

Integrity

Each tendon transferred should have a single function. Tenodesis to a tendon that has a communal function will produce satisfactory results, whereas tenodesis to tendons with separate functions will not. An example of the former is the Bridle procedure. An attempt to restore dorsiflexion and balance the foot is performed by transfer of the posterior tibial tendon through the interosseus membrane and creation of an insertion on the dorsum of the midfoot. Tenodesis is also performed between the transferred posterior tibial tendon and both the anterior tibial tendon and an anteriorly rerouted peroneus longus.[14] Although multiple attachments are made, all act for a balanced, concerted motion. Another important aspect to the principle of integrity is that multiple attachments from a single transferred tendon must all be able to achieve the same excursion. Failure to adhere to this results in the production of a checkrein effect.

Tensioning

The tension at which a tendon transfer is set is intimately related to the strength of the muscle transfer and therefore has direct bearing on that principle of tendon transfers. The proper tension to set a tendon transfer has been a source of controversy since the inception of these techniques.[5] Some experts opine that the musculotendinous unit should be placed on maximum passive stretch before fixation to bone, whereas others feel that the tension should be closer to the midrange between maximal tension and complete laxity.

A muscle fiber responds differently under passive as opposed to active conditions. When a muscle fiber is passively lengthened it acts much like an elastic band: The more the fiber is stretched, the more tension is realized until the point of failure (rupture). However, this linear relationship is not maintained when we look at the active tension able to be generated by a muscle in relationship to changes to the resting length of muscle.

Those espousing the midrange of muscle tension cite the Blix curve as support. The Blix curve describes the close relationship between the starting length of a muscle fiber and its ability to generate tension in response to nerve stimulation (**Fig. 1**).[15] When a fiber is at or slightly longer than its resting length, maximum active tension is realized. As a fiber's starting length decreases from its resting length (to the left along the length–tension curve) tension production decreases. Similarly, when the fiber's starting length is increased from the point of maximum tension

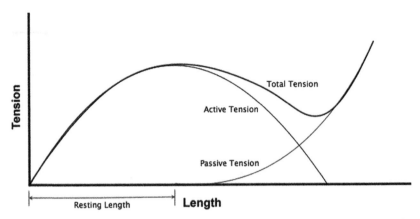

Fig. 1. Blix curve. Curve describing the length tension relationship or the musculotendinous unit.

generation (ie, stretched, to the right of the curve) active tension production again decreases. The same relationship holds true for the gross muscle.

At the histologic level, the relationship between length and tension generated is explained by the amount of actin–myosin overlap within the sarcomere. At the resting length nearly all of the myosin heads are in contact with actin (**Fig. 2**A). When the muscle fiber is stimulated to fire maximal tension is generated because of this optimal overlap. As the muscle lengthens beyond its resting length this overlap starts to diminish (see **Fig. 2**B) and as a result the amount of tension able to be generated wanes. If the starting length is less than the resting length, the myosin is not able to optimally progress along the actin filament and less tension is realized.

The Blix curve provides a good graphical representation of the effects of muscle length on contraction. One shortcoming, however, is that it does not account for the phenomenon that, as a muscle nears the end of its excursion, its ability to generate tension is diminished by the passive tension being developed in its antagonists. The length–tension relationship suggests that, under most normal movement conditions, the body, through either motor control or biomechanical strategies, attempts to optimize muscle length so that maximal force, torque, and power can be produced.

Those suggesting that the transferred motor unit be placed under tension claim that it adjusts with time to maximize functional response. Until recently, however, there has been no basic science to corroborate or refute this. Using an animal model in which a tendon transfer was performed placing the musculotendinous unit on tension, Takahashi and colleagues[16] demonstrated that there is an initial increase in the sarcomere number within the muscle transferred. This increase is followed by a decrease in sarcomere number and eventually an increase in the tendon length (**Fig. 3**). This complex adaptation to tensioning occurring during tendon transfer suggests that the musculotendinous unit has at least some ability to adjust overtensioning to maximize the functional response.

Muscles with longer fiber lengths are able to sustain their force of contraction over a greater range of motion than those with short fiber lengths. The length–tension curves of short muscles generally rise and fall quickly, whereas those of longer muscles have a more broad curve.[17] For this reason, a short-bellied muscle with short excursion is not suited to replace a strap-type, long excursion muscle.[1]

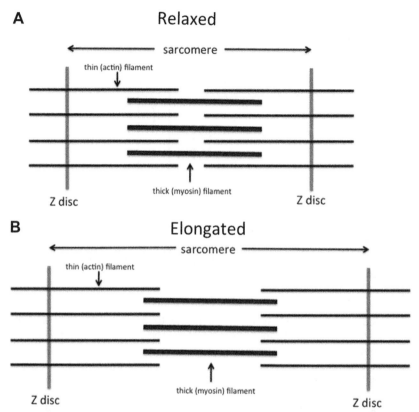

Fig. 2. At the histologic level, the relationship between length and tension generated is explained by the amount of actin-myosin overlap within the sarcomere. (*A*) At resting length, nearly all of the myosin heads are in contact with actin. When the muscle fiber is stimulated to fire maximal tension is generated because of this optimal overlap. (*B*) As the muscle lengthens beyond its resting length, this overlap starts to diminish and as a result the amount of tension able to be generated wanes. If the starting length is less than the resting length, the myosin is not able to optimally progress along the actin filament and less tension is realized.

Formation of a Stable Bone–Tendon Interface

Stable attachment of the tendon to bone is requisite to the long-term proper functioning of a tendon transfer. The study of the development of the transferred tendon–bone interface has been ongoing for over 70 years.

Initial studies

Kernwein and colleagues[18] was among the early groups to look at the histologic maturation of tendon transfers to bone. This group described the process as "ossification of the tendon,"[18] It was almost another 20 years before the subject was seriously studied again by Whiston and Walmsley.[19] Just after the publication of this work, Forward and Cowan[20] described the process as starting with formation of connective tissue sleeve which then progressed to invasion of fibroblasts into tendon.

Most recently, Rodeo's group has enhanced our understanding of the maturation of tendon transfers to bone. Although it utilized animal models of anterior cruciate

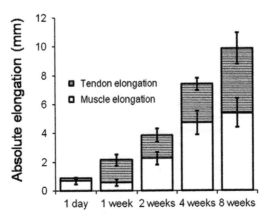

Fig. 3. Tendon–muscle elongation. Graph depicting the in vivo animal results of Takahashi and colleagues,[16] which demonstrate the adaptation of both muscle and tendon after transfer under tension. (*From* Takahashi M, Ward SR, Marchuk LL, et al. Asynchronous muscle and tendon adaptation after surgical tensioning procedures. J Bone Joint Surg Am 2010;92: 664; with permission.[16])

ligament reconstruction, their work is applicable to any situation where there is establishment of a stable tendon–bone interface. Their work has identified 3 phases in this process. The first is the formation of fibrovascular tissue at the tendon–bone interface (**Fig. 4**A) This occurs in the first 2 weeks after the tendon transplant is performed. In this phase, there is a vascular, highly cellular fibrous interface between the tendon and bone. Between 2 and 12 weeks, a thin seam of new bone lines the bone tunnel. The tissue at the interface shows increased production of matrix with a decrease in vascularity in comparison with the 2-week specimens. There is occasional continuity of collagen fibers from bone to the tendon (see **Fig. 4**B) twelve weeks after transfer, there is increased maturation of the interface tissue with fibers starting to align themselves along the direction of pull of the tendon. Twenty-six weeks after tendon transfer into bone, there is increased alignment of the collagen fibers along the direction of pull of the tendon throughout the length of the tendon. There is also remodeling of the trabecular bone surrounding the tendon (see **Fig. 4**C) The last phase is maturation of tendon–bone interface.[21]

It seems that approximately 3 months is required after tendon transfer for a stable bone–tendon interface to be formed. Rodeo's group performed biomechanical testing to evaluate the strength of the tendon–bone interface while this process was ongoing. During the first 8 weeks after tendon implantation, all specimens failed by pullout of the tendon at the bone–tendon interface. By 12 weeks, the interface had strengthened so that failure occurred at the tendon clamp or in the tendon midsubstance. There was no further functional maturation of this interface past 12 weeks.[21]

Tendon Anchoring

A number of different methods have been successfully used to secure tendon to bone. Early methods of fixation included passing the tendon through a bone tunnel and then suturing it back upon itself. This requires an adequate length of tendon and a location at which it is possible to turn the tendon back upon itself. Another method that can be utilized when it is difficult to suture the tendon upon itself is to pass the tendon through a bone tunnel and secure it to a button on the skin.[22] A number of

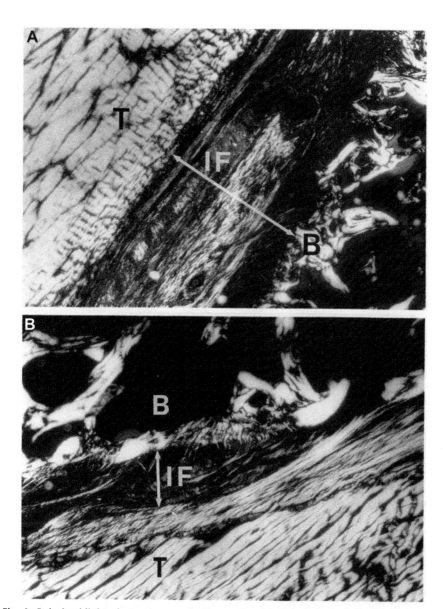

Fig. 4. Polarized light photomicrographs illustrating the progression of bone–tendon healing with time. (*A*) The first phase, which is seen in during the first 2 weeks after tendon implantation into bone, involves the formation of fibrovascular tissue at the tendon–bone interface. (*B*) After the first 2 weeks after implantation, a thin seam of new bone lining the tunnel begins to be seen. The occasional continuity of collagen fibers from bone to the tendon, becomes more prevalent by 12 weeks. (*C*) By 26 weeks, there is increased alignment of the collagen fibers along the direction of pull of the tendon throughout the length of the tendon. Remodeling of the trabecular bone surrounding the tendon is also seen. B, bone; IF, interface; T, tendon. (From Poppen N. Soft-tissue lesions of the shoulder. In Chapman M, Madison M, editors. Operative orthopaedics. Philadelphia: Lippincott; 1988. p. 745; with permission.[38])

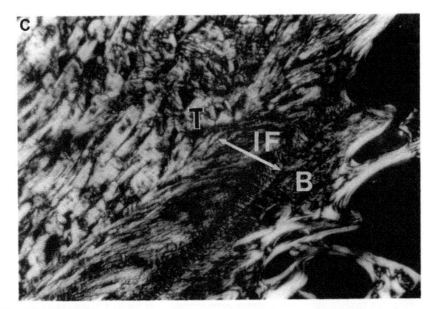

Fig. 4. (*continued*)

commercial devices have also been developed to strengthen fixation or provide fixation alternatives when tendon length is limited. These include staples,[23] spiked washers,[24] bone anchors,[25] soft tissue interference screws,[26] and adjustable suture suspension within bone.[27]

Soft tissue interference screws were originally constructed from titanium. These were found to have the unacceptable complication of occasionally lacerating the tendon graft.[28] Bioabsorbable screws demonstrate adequate fixation with minimal damage to the graft. These screws have been fashioned from poly-L-lactic acid and bone dowels. These have become the choice of surgeons using soft tissue interference screws in recent years. Less traumatic, nonabsorbable screws have also been fashioned from polyetheretherketone and are now commercially available.[29]

Scranton and colleagues[30] looked at suture anchor fixation in cadaveric bone. Differences in insertion technique yielded varying results. Anchors composed of plastic failed at the eyelet. They concluded that if suture anchors are used at least 2 should be placed for each anchor point.[30] The angle of suture anchor insertion also influences pullout strength. Burkhart showed that the "deadman's angle" allows the threads of the anchor and the structure of the surrounding bone to combine to maximize pullout strength of these devices. This angle of the insertion is such that the inserted point of the bone anchor is canted approximately 45° toward the direction of pull of the tendon.[31,32]

Sullivan and colleagues[33] compared the strength of suture anchor fixation to sewing the tendon to itself when transferring the flexor digitorum longus to the medial navicular. They demonstrated that the mean load to failure was nearly identical for each group.[33] Although use of suture anchor fixation requires less tendon length, there is a much greater cost of using these devices compared with simply suturing the tendon back upon itself after passage through a bone tunnel. A similar experimental design was employed by Sabonghy and colleagues,[26] but using soft tissue interference screws rather than suture anchors. This group found that sewing the tendon to itself was stronger than using a soft tissue interference screw, but both provided enough strength at the bone–tendon interface to counteract physiologic forces encountered by tendons.

A recent study comparing the strength of fixation using a bone anchor versus that of soft tissue interference screws was evaluated in an in vitro model of the split anterior tendon transfer.[34] The soft tissue interference screw fixation was significantly stronger, but it is unknown whether this translates into a clinical difference. A study with a similar design looking at fixation strength for an autograft lateral ankle ligament reconstruction showed that the soft tissue interference screw was significantly stronger in fixing the tendon to bone than bone anchors. The values obtained for the soft tissue interference screws seem to be greater than the values for load to failure of the native anterior talofibular ligament.[35]

The frequently asked question of how large a tunnel should be used when soft tissue interference screws are employed was addressed by Louden and colleagues.[36] In this study, pilot hole diameter was varied for 2 different sizes of interference screws to determine which provided better fixation strength. The authors noted that there was a significant difference in pullout strength between 7 and 5 mm screws, but pilot hole size did not influence the pullout strength for a given screw size. Greater than adequate fixation was obtained with both screw sizes irrespective of pilot hole size even in elderly cadaveric bone.

Location

Classic teaching has been that tendon transfers will heal better to a raw bleeding cancellous surface than to intact cortical bone. Nowhere is this more evident than in the belief that for proper healing rotator cuff repairs must be secured into a cancellous trough at the greater tuberosity of the humerus.[37,38] The exact rationale for this teaching is not known, but likely arose from the belief that the interface that forms between a tendon and cancellous bone is biomechanically superior to that formed between a tendon and cortical bone. St Pierre and colleagues[39] tested this assumption in an in vivo animal model of rotator cuff repair. They compared the biomechanical properties of infraspinatus repairs affixed with a cortical trough to those repaired directly to cancellous bone. Interestingly, there was no difference in the strength of repairs in the load to failure, energy to failure or stiffness between the 2 groups at 6 and 12 weeks after the repair.[39]

Biologics and Physiologic Factors

The study of biologics and biologic response modifiers in relation to tendon transfers is in its infancy. Although a number of different biologics have been investigated the number of studies performed is low. Some of the substances studied are not available commercially but have been included for completeness.

Bone morphogenetic proteins are growth factors that induce bone formation in tissues with the capacity to do so.[40] An in vivo animal study has demonstrated that bone morphogenetic protein-2 is able to augment tendon healing to bone.[41] This study was performed in a two-stage model in which an ossicle was generated within the tendon to be transferred and this tendon–ossicle complex was then fixed to the recipient site. With this model, higher ultimate load to failure values were observed after healing. However, it is unclear whether such a two-stage approach could be practically adopted in clinical practice.

Receptor activator of nuclear factor-κB ligand is a major stimulatory factor for osteoclast formation in cells of the monocyte lineage. It also has direct catabolic effects on bone and has been shown to reduce bone density, volume and strength.[42] Because of these findings, it was thought that the receptor activator of nuclear factor-κB ligand would diminish the tendon bone interface. However, its addition did not decrease the histologic or biomechanical properties of the bone–tendon interface compared with control specimens. Osteoprotegerin is a soluble receptor antagonist to the receptor activator of nuclear factor-κB. Because it antagonizes osteoclast formation, it augments the maturation of the bone–tendon interface.[43]

Platelet concentrates also modulate tendon-to-bone healing. Addition of platelet concentrate alone to hamstring anterior cruciate ligament reconstruction led to uniform magnetic resonance imaging evidence of graft incorporation within a bone tunnel at 6 months that was significantly improved over a control group. However, no functionally statistical differences in the groups were found.[44]

One group has tested a magnesium-based bone adhesive for repairing flexor tendons to bone in an animal model. They found that the initial biomechanical properties of these repairs are improved with the adhesive, but in vivo use led to a decrease in the strength of the repair.[45] Presently, the use of these adhesives cannot be recommended.

Nonsteroidal Anti-Inflammatory Drugs

The effect of nonsteroidal anti-inflammatory drug (NSAID) use on tendon–bone healing has been investigated.[46–48] Most recently, Dimmen and colleagues[47] showed that the development of a strong interface relative to untreated control animals was delayed by NSAIDs. In the study animals, 3 groups were tested for strength to pullout. There were 2 study groups that received either parecoxib or indomethacin after Achilles tendon transplant into the tibia. The control group did not receive any NSAID. Both experimental groups showed significantly diminished interfaces relative to the control group.[47]

Nicotine

Although the detrimental effects of nicotine on fracture healing and joint fusion have been well described, little is known about its effect on the healing of soft tissues such as tendon and ligament. In an in vivo model of healing of rotator cuff to bone, Galatz and colleagues[49] demonstrated that the rotator cuff attachment of animals exposed to nicotine had decreased maximum stress and maximum force relative to those in the control group. They also demonstrated that cellular proliferation and type I collagen expression was lower in the nicotine-treated animals relative to controls. Inflammation persisted longer in the nicotine-treated animals. The authors surmised that these findings may at least partly explain the inferior biomechanical properties demonstrated by the nicotine-treated groups.[49]

Immobilization/Mobilization

Tendons and their entheses respond to mechanical changes in their environment. In general, increased loads across these structures lead to increases in their tensile modulus, while decreases in applied stress causes a diminution in their mechanical properties.

Studies on early loading of tendon grafts have been contradictory. One previous study demonstrated that the strength of graft integration of rabbit anterior cruciate ligament repairs was impaired in animals allowed unlimited cage activity.[50] Another showed that early exercise compromised healing of an animal rotator cuff repair model. However, Thomopoulos and colleagues[51] have subsequently demonstrated that muscle loading after canine flexor tendon repair improved the biomechanical properties compared with animals whose repairs went unloaded. Most recently, Bedi and colleagues[52] showed that early delayed application of cyclic axial loads increased load to failure, new bone formation, tissue mineral content and density at the tendon bone interface. The load to failure was highest in animals that had daily applied loads started 4 days postoperatively.[52] It is difficult to compare these studies because different animal models and tendon surgeries were examined.

SUMMARY

Tendon transfers are powerful procedures that have demonstrated the ability to restore substantial function to appropriately selected patients. However, there are important procedural considerations and inherent limitations to acknowledge before the use of these techniques. It is imperative to understand the patient's needs and goals and match them with the appropriate procedure. Tendon transfers are optimally performed within a healthy soft tissue bed, across mobile joints, and using proper donor tissue characteristics (strength, excursion, expendability, direction of pull, phase, and integrity). Appropriate tensioning and insertion points must be chosen. Finally, perioperative care should include appropriate immobilization, subsequent rehabilitation, analgesics, and avoidance of nicotine. A thorough understanding and proper implementation of these concepts will optimize the outcome when surgeons use tendon transfers in the treatment of musculoskeletal conditions.

REFERENCES

1. Peabody C. Tendon transposition. J Bone Joint Surg Am 1938;20:193.
2. Nicoladoni C. Nachtrag zum Pes Calcaneus und zur Transplantation die Peronealsehnen. Arch f Klin Chirurgie 1882;27:660.
3. Erlacher PJ. The development of tendon surgery in Germany; a review of the history and an evaluation of the treatment. Instr Course Lect 1986;13:110.
4. Herndon CH. Tendon transplantation at the knee and foot. Instr Course Lect 1961; 18:145.
5. Mayer L. The physiologic method of tendon transplantation. I. Historical, anatomy and physiology of tendons. Surg Gynecol Obstet 1916;22.
6. Hansen S. Functional Reconstruction of the Foot and Ankle. Philadelphia: Lippincott, Williams and Wilkins; 2000.
7. Young C. Operative treatment of pes planus. Surg Gyn Obst 1939;68:1099.
8. Makin M. Translocation of the flexor pollicis longus tendon to restore opposition. J Bone Joint Surg Br 1967;49:458.
9. Lin CH, Lin YT, Yeh JT, et al. Free functioning muscle transfer for lower extremity posttraumatic composite structure and functional defect. Plast Reconstr Surg 2007; 119:2118.
10. Chuang DC. Functioning free muscle transplantation for brachial plexus injury. Clin Orthop Relat Res 1995;314:104.
11. Henderson M. Results following tenosuspension operations for habitual dislocation of the shoulder. J Bone Joint Surg Am 1935;17:978.
12. Levitt RL, Canale ST, Cooke AJ Jr, et al. The role of foot surgery in progressive neuromuscular disorders in children. J Bone Joint Surg Am 1973;55:1396.
13. Close JR, Todd FN. The phasic activity of the muscles of the lower extremity and the effect of tendon transfer. J Bone Joint Surg Am 1959;41-A:189.
14. Rodriguez RP. The bridle procedure in the treatment of paralysis of the foot. Foot Ankle 1992;13:63.
15. Blix M. Die Lange und die Spannung des Muskels. Skand Arch Physiol 1895;5:173–206.

16. Takahashi M, Ward SR, Marchuk LL, et al. Asynchronous muscle and tendon adaptation after surgical tensioning procedures. J Bone Joint Surg Am 2010;92:664.

17. Peljovich A, Ratner JA, Marino J. Update of the physiology and biomechanics of tendon transfer surgery. J Hand Surg Am 2010 35:1365–9.

18. Kernwein G. Tendon implantations to bone: a study of the factors affecting tendon-bone union as determined by the tensile strength. Ann Surg 1941;113:1103.

19. Whiston TB, Walmsley R. Some observations on the reactions of bone and tendon after tunnelling of bone and insertion of tendon. J Bone Joint Surg Br 1960;42-B:377.

20. Forward AD, Cowan RJ. Experimental suture of tendon to bone. Surg Forum 1960;11:458.

21. Rodeo SA, Arnoczky SP, Torzilli PA, et al. Tendon-healing in a bone tunnel. A biomechanical and histological study in the dog. J Bone Joint Surg Am 1993;75: 1795.

22. Key JA. Fixation of tendons, ligaments and bone by Bunnell's pull-out wire suture. Ann Surg 1946;123:656.

23. Goh JC, Lee PY, Lee EH, et al. Biomechanical study on tibialis posterior tendon transfers. Clin Orthop Relat Res 1995;319:297.

24. Straight CB, France EP, Paulos LE, et al. Soft tissue fixation to bone. A biomechanical analysis of spiked washers. Am J Sports Med 1994;22:339.

25. Myerson MS, Cohen I, Uribe J. An easy way of tensioning and securing a tendon to bone. Foot Ankle Int 2002;23:753.

26. Sabonghy EP, Wood RM, Ambrose CG, et al. Tendon transfer fixation: comparing a tendon to tendon technique vs. bioabsorbable interference-fit screw fixation. Foot Ankle Int 2003;24:260.

27. Bluman EM. Technique tip: suture suspension of tendons. Foot Ankle Int 2007; 28:854.

28. McGuire DA, Barber FA, Elrod BF, et al. Bioabsorbable interference screws for graft fixation in anterior cruciate ligament reconstruction. Arthroscopy 1999;15:463.

29. Nho SJ, Provencher MT, Seroyer ST, et al. Bioabsorbable anchors in glenohumeral shoulder surgery. Arthroscopy 2009;25:788.

30. Scranton PE Jr, Lawhon SM, McDermott JE. Bone suture anchor fixation in the lower extremity: a review of insertion principles and a comparative biomechanical evaluation. Foot Ankle Int 2005;26:516.

31. Burkhart SS, Lo IKY, Brady PC. Burkhart's view of the shoulder: a cowboy's guide to advanced shoulder arthroscopy. Philadelphia: Lippincott Williams & Wilkins; 2006.

32. Strauss E, Frank D, Kubiak E, et al. The effect of the angle of suture anchor insertion on fixation failure at the tendon-suture interface after rotator cuff repair: deadman's angle revisited. Arthroscopy 2009;25:597.

33. Sullivan RJ, Gladwell HA, Aronow MS, et al. An in vitro study comparing the use of suture anchors and drill hole fixation for flexor digitorum longus transfer to the navicular. Foot Ankle Int 2006;27:363.

34. Nunez-Pereira S, Pacha-Vicente D, Llusa-Perez M, et al. Tendon transfer fixation in the foot and ankle: a biomechanical study. Foot Ankle Int 2009;30:1207.

35. Jeys L, Korrosis S, Stewart T, et al. Bone anchors or interference screws? A biomechanical evaluation for autograft ankle stabilization. Am J Sports Med 2004;32: 1651.

36. Louden KW, Ambrose CG, Beaty SG, et al. Tendon transfer fixation in the foot and ankle: a biomechanical study evaluating two sizes of pilot holes for bioabsorbable screws. Foot Ankle Int 2003;24:67.

37. Shoulder and elbow injuries. In: Crenshaw AH, Daugherty K, Campbell WC, editors. Campbell's operative orthopaedics. 8th edition. St Louis: Mosby Year Book; 1992. p. 5 v.

38. Poppen N. Soft-tissue lesions of the shoulder. In: Chapman M, Madison M, editors. Operative orthopaedics. Philadelphia: Lippincott; 1988. p. 745.

39. St Pierre P, Olson EJ, Elliott JJ, et al. Tendon-healing to cortical bone compared with healing to a cancellous trough. A biomechanical and histological evaluation in goats. J Bone Joint Surg Am 1995;77:1858.

40. Gautschi OP, Frey SP, Zellweger R. Bone morphogenetic proteins in clinical applications. Aust N Z J Surg 2007;77:626.

41. Hashimoto Y, Yoshida G, Toyoda H, et al. Generation of tendon-to-bone interface "enthesis" with use of recombinant BMP-2 in a rabbit model. J Orthop Res 2007;25: 1415.

42. Kostenuik PJ. Osteoprotegerin and RANKL regulate bone resorption, density, geometry and strength. Curr Opin Pharmacol 2005;5:618.

43. Rodeo SA, Kawamura S, Ma CB, et al. The effect of osteoclastic activity on tendon-to-bone healing: an experimental study in rabbits. J Bone Joint Surg Am 2007;89: 2250.

44. Orrego M, Larrain C, Rosales J, et al. Effects of platelet concentrate and a bone plug on the healing of hamstring tendons in a bone tunnel. Arthroscopy 2008;24:1373.

45. Thomopoulos S, Zampiakis E, Das R, et al. Use of a magnesium-based bone adhesive for flexor tendon-to-bone healing. J Hand Surg Am 2009;34:1066.

46. Cohen DB, Kawamura S, Ehteshami JR, et al. Indomethacin and celecoxib impair rotator cuff tendon-to-bone healing. Am J Sports Med 2006;34:362.

47. Dimmen S, Nordsletten L, Engebretsen L, et al. The effect of parecoxib and indomethacin on tendon-to-bone healing in a bone tunnel: an experimental study in rats. J Bone Joint Surg Br 2009;91:259.

48. Ferry ST, Dahners LE, Afshari HM, et al. The effects of common anti-inflammatory drugs on the healing rat patellar tendon. Am J Sports Med 2007;35:1326.

49. Galatz LM, Silva MJ, Rothermich SY, et al. Nicotine delays tendon-to-bone healing in a rat shoulder model. J Bone Joint Surg Am 2006;88:2027.

50. Sakai H, Fukui N, Kawakami A, et al. Biological fixation of the graft within bone after anterior cruciate ligament reconstruction in rabbits: effects of the duration of postoperative immobilization. J Orthop Sci 2000;5:43.

51. Thomopoulos S, Zampiakis E, Das R, et al. The effect of muscle loading on flexor tendon-to-bone healing in a canine model. J Orthop Res 2008;26:1611.

52. Bedi A, Kovacevic D, Fox AJ, et al. Effect of early and delayed mechanical loading on tendon-to-bone healing after anterior cruciate ligament reconstruction. J Bone Joint Surg Am 2010;92:2387–401.

Tendon Transfers for Equinovarus Deformity in Adults and Children

Christopher Bibbo, DO, DPM[a],*, Samarjit S. Jaglan, MD[b]

KEYWORDS

- Tendon transfer • Foot deformities • Equinovarus deformity
- Pediatrics • Adults

Strictly defined, an equinovarus foot deformity positions the foot and ankle in both equinus and varus. However, triplanar joint axes, coupled joint motion, and secondary contractures result in deformity within in the sagittal, transverse, and frontal planes. This complex deformity pattern results in a foot and ankle posture that makes it extremely difficult to ambulate correctly, stand at ease, or even allow appropriate orthotic/prosthetic fitting (**Fig. 1A**). In a series of 177 patients who sustained hemiplegic stroke, the positive impact of tendon transfer surgery for equinovarus deformity included improved foot position, a faster gait, and improved propulsion.[1] This article describes the etiologies, evaluation, and operative management of equinovarus deformity in adults and pediatric populations by tendon transfer and ancillary soft tissue releases.

TENDON TRANSFERS FOR EQUINOVARUS DEFORMITY IN ADULTS

A complete review of the protagonist-antagonist relationships and electrophysiologic activities of the lower extremity musculoskeletal units during gait is beyond the scope of this article. However, in the equinovarus foot and ankle, it should be reinforced that the primary deforming forces include the posterior tibial tendon (PTT), the gastrocnemius-soleus complex, the flexor hallucis longus tendon (FHL), and the flexor digitorum longus tendon (FDL) (in decreasing order of magnitude). These motor units overpower their antagonists, either because of weakening or complete loss of the latter. Secondary soft-tissue contractures then maintain or even exacerbate the deformity.

In addition to equinus, a substantial amount of varus deformity can develop through the ankle and subtalar joints, and to a lesser extent through the midfoot distal

[a] Foot & Ankle Section, Department of Orthopaedics, Marshfield Clinic, Marshfield, WI 54449, USA
[b] Pediatric Orthopaedic Section, Department of Orthopaedics, Marshfield Clinic, Marshfield, WI 54449, USA
* Corresponding author.
E-mail address: bibbo.christopher@marshfieldclinic.org

Foot Ankle Clin N Am 16 (2011) 401–418
doi:10.1016/j.fcl.2011.07.001
1083-7515/11/$ – see front matter © 2011 Elsevier Inc. All rights reserved.

foot.theclinics.com

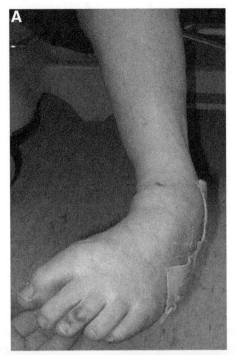

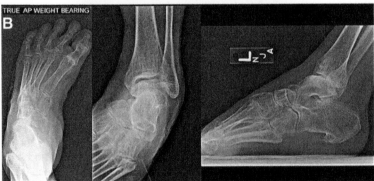

Fig. 1. (*A*) Posture of the equinovarus foot. Note the lateral column overload from shoe pressure and limited attempted weight bearing. (*B*) Radiographs of a mild-moderate equinovarus foot. Note the varus and adducted position of the foot, overcoverage of the talonavicular joint, ankle equinus, heel varus, and "stacking" of the metatarsals.

to the transverse tarsal joint. Additionally, both the equinus and varus deformities may be static, dynamic, or combinations thereof, depending on the etiology of the deformity. As discussed later, the time course at which these etiologies progress into an equinovarus deformity vary. Compounding the clinical presentation, a lower motor neuron (LMN) or upper motor neuron lesion may occur in the face of a preexisting neurologic condition. These lesions may result in secondary deformities, the natural history of which needs to be considered in order to provide long-lasting deformity correction without compromising existing lower extremity power. Thus, the history and physical exam, albeit a challenge, is paramount, enabling the surgeon to develop an optimal surgical plan. Despite the inherent challenges in the treatment of the equinovarus limb, reconstructive efforts are quite rewarding, whether it is because patients can simply wear shoes and heal recalcitrant wounds or because they can stand, transfer, and ambulate.

Patient Evaluation

Several critical pieces of information are necessary to guide the surgeon through the clinical decision-making process, as well as through the immediate perioperative period and long-term follow-up.

The first issue that the surgeon must consider is the etiology behind the deformity along with its natural history. Is the result a primarily a flaccid or spastic deformity? Where in the natural history of the condition the patient presents must also be ascertained. Despite equinovarus being the most common foot deformity after hemiplegic cerebral vascular accident (CVA), many patients may reacquire a relatively plantigrade foot posture over the first 6 months following the CVA and may not necessarily require extensive surgical intervention. Additionally, post-CVA patients may exhibit body neglect rather than flaccid paralysis. In comparison, patients with traumatic brain injury (TBI) demonstrate a course of improvement that may last more than 20 months. In patients with LMN injuries from trauma, initial neurologic deficits should be evaluated with baseline electrodiagnostic testing. Complete nerve transections (especially open injuries) should be treated with immediate nerve repair/reconstruction. The discovery of incomplete injuries should be followed by serial electrodiagnostic testing every 3 to 4 months to assess recovery. Recently, in a series of 62 patients with complete traumatic peroneal nerve injury and dropfoot, improved results were found when simultaneous posterior-to-anterior tendon transfer was combined with nerve reconstruction at a single operative setting performed at 3 to 4 months postinjury.[2] However, we have observed patients with incomplete injuries developing partial return of motor nerve function sufficient for functional bracing, eliminating the need for tendon transfer as late as 24 months postinjury. Thus, careful follow-up and evaluation of the patients is paramount, and treatment plans need to be individualized to the pattern of nerve recovery and patient needs.

The second general item that must be carefully evaluated in the patient with equinovarus foot deformity is the existence of secondary soft tissue and joint contractures (see **Fig. 1**B; **Fig. 2**). Secondary contractures may result from a primary spastic condition, or from the normal contracture of a muscle or muscle group that is unopposed by flaccid antagonists. These contractures may be reflected in either one or both components of the equinovarus deformity and are usually a progressive process. The surgeon must be able to anticipate the necessary releases of secondary contractures and incorporate them into the operative plan (**Box 1**). It is the corresponding author's experience that in the early period (1–5 y) after a neurologic deficit resulting in an LMN injury, secondary (acquired) contractures are less likely to be evident and, if present, may be supple. However, 10 to 15 years after the neurologic event, acquired contractures are invariably present, fixed, and involve both soft tissue and joints.

The third general consideration that the surgeon must evaluate is the effect of an acquired equinovarus deformity on the neurovascular structures. Chronic, progressive deformities also result in relative "shortening" of the neurovascular structures. Acute deformity correction in the severe equinovarus foot may thereby result in substantial lengthening of the neurovascular structures. If the surgeon anticipates any

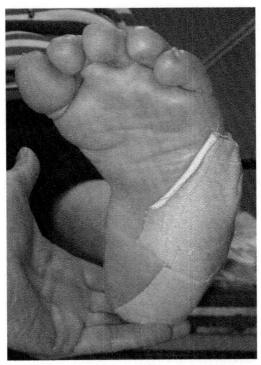

Fig. 2. Attitude of equinovarus foot; primary and secondary soft-tissue and joint contractures are evident (see **Box 1**).

detrimental neurovascular effects from acute deformity correction, then gradual soft tissue lengthening techniques should be considered before tendon transfers (**Fig. 3**).

Finally, a global assessment of the patient must be performed with regard to the severity of the inciting event (eg, CVA, TBI), the patient's potential for use of the proposed tendon transfer, and the specific needs of the patient. Additionally, the patient's physical and cognitive abilities and the available medical/community resources should be assessed to determine the most appropriate and effective method to meet the goals of the surgery.

Operative Principles

The general guidelines for addressing the equinovarus deformity with tendon transfers have been previously addressed in this issue but bear reinforcement. First, transferred tendons lose one grade of strength after transfer due to alterations in the natural course of the tendon (decreased mechanical advantage) and unavoidable weakening from surgical manipulation. In order to provide a functional tendon transfer, the muscle/tendon unit to be transferred should posses a minimum strength grade of 4/5. Transfers of tendons with less power ultimately result in a functional tenodesis, which may allow for adequate positioning but lacks dynamic function. Second, tendons to be transferred should be in the same phase during the gait cycle; however, the muscle/tendon units being transferred for equinovarus are all out-of-phase. In order to maximize functional potential of these out-of-phase transfers, retraining in physical therapy is mandatory. Third, to maximize power, transferred

---

Box 1
Common primary and secondary contractures in the equinovarus deformity

Ankle joint: Varus deformity with deltoid contracture, lateral ankle ligament insufficiency; contracted posterior ankle capsule and medial fibro-osseous tunnels.

Subtalar joint: Supination deformity with tight interosseous ligament and medial capsule; lax cervical ligament.

Transverse tarsal joint: Talonavicular with medial/plantar capsular contracture and "overcoverage"; calcaneocuboid joint with tight medial capsule and interosseous ligaments.

Naviculocuneiform and tarsometatarsal joints: Contracted plantar medial ligamentous structures and spring ligament complex.

Posterior tibial tendon: Main deforming force in primary and acquired equinovarus.

Tibialis anterior tendon: Contributes to varus position in spastic conditions.

Flexor hallucis longus and flexor digitorum longus tendons: Tendon sheaths and tendons; possible muscle belly fibrosis; zones involved include leg, ankle, foot.

Gastrocnemius-soleus complex: Contracture of muscle, fascia, aponeurosis, and Achilles tendon; may result in heel varus in addition to ankle equinus.

Deep posterior crural fascia: Constricts extrinsic muscles and tendons, tethers posterior neurovascular bundle; expansion of deep crural fascia intimate with peri-Achilles fascia and lacinate ligament.

Abductor hallucis muscle and fascia: Contracture contributes to hindfoot and midfoot varus with associated cavus posture.

Adductor hallucis-calcaneal fascial band: Must be released in extreme secondary contracture of the abductor hallucis muscle fascia.

Plantar fascia: Contracture findings similar to abductor hallucis.

Tarsal tunnel: Lacinate ligament and its expansions; prophylactic release in advanced deformity may prevent neural compromise.

Skin and subcutaneous tissues: Severe, chronic deformity may result in nonpliable cutaneous structures that may prove to be a tether and compromise wound healing.

---

tendons should have as straight a course as possible. The path of transfer must be free of obstacles and, if transferred through an aperture, the window of passage should be wide and allow easy gliding and maximum excursion of the tendon. Fourth, deforming forces (muscle-tendon units, altered mechanical axis) must be neutralized, minimized, or weakened. Otherwise, a component of the deformity is likely to recur. Finally, the limb must be stable. Unstable joints must be stabilized by ligamentous procedures, osteotomy, or arthrodesis. These procedures may be performed simultaneously or in a staged fashion. Osteotomies that greatly translate the mechanical axis (eg, a calcaneal V osteotomy) may be less desirable than an arthrodesis.

Specific Operative Techniques

Isolated posterior tibial tendon transfer
The isolated PTT transfer is a relatively straightforward technique that attempts to restore ankle dorsiflexion via direct relocation of the insertion of the PTT to the midfoot, first described by Watkins and colleagues[3] in 1954 for treatment of equinovarus deformity secondary to poliomyelitis. This technique is most successful when some active function of the medial dorsiflexors (tibialis anterior, extensor

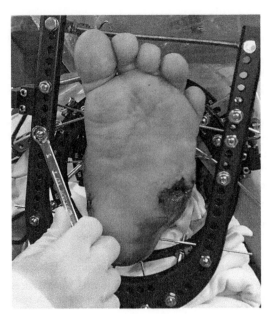

Fig. 3. Application of a circular fine-wire external fixator for severe equinovarus. Initial soft tissue releases are performed, and gradual correction is performed before tendon transfers. Lateral ulceration and underlying osteomyelitis treated at first-stage surgery.

hallucis longus) remains or flaccid paralysis of ankle dorsiflexion is easily passively corrected, or the varus component of equinovarus is purely dynamic (minimal to no acquired medial fixed varus). In essence, the isolated transfer of the PTT acts as a compliment to an active but overpowered tibialis anterior, providing a functional lateral ankle dorsiflexor. In all instances, the equinus must be neutralized by addressing the gastrocnemius-soleus complex. On occasion, the deep posterior leg compartment (particularly the FHL) must also be released (eg, posttraumatic fibrosis/ossification, post deep-compartment syndrome contracture).

The patient is placed supine and the leg is positioned to allow easy access to posterior medial ankle structures and the dorsum of the foot. General anesthesia is preferred with neuromuscular blockade. A thigh tourniquet is used, and chlorhexidine skin prep is preferred.[4] Proximal indwelling pain catheters may be used. A long posterior medial incision is placed directly behind the medial malleolus. The PTT is identified and dissected distally to its insertion. The tendon is released from the navicular only, yet harvesting as much length as possible, preferably with a periosteal cuff that can be tubularized. Proximally, through the same or a separate proximal incision, the PTT is followed to the inferior edge of the deep crural fascia, which is split and released. This is often contracted and tethers the tendon. The free end of the PTT is tagged with a sturdy suture and the distal end tubularized as necessary.

Next, an anterior incision is made over the lateral from the midfoot (navicular-cuneiform level), extending proximally to above the level of the syndesmosis, avoiding damage to the syndesmosis and the perforating peroneal artery. The goal of this is identification of the thinner interosseous membrane (IOM). A generous aperture is created in the IOM to allow passage of the PTT and any low-lying muscle belly that may travel through the membrane. A long clamp is used to widen the aperture; finger dissection on the posterior IOM is often wise, using the finger to sweep away muscular attachments (FHL) as well as small vascular branches that may lead to hematoma. The PTT remains along a fairly in-line course when passing through the aperture. The tag stitch on the PTT is then grasped with the clamp, and the PTT is passed through the IOM from posterior to anterior. Passing an additional clamp from anterior to posterior, opening the clamp jaws, and then advancing the posterior clamp and tendon through the IOM into the anterior leg is helpful if the compartments are tight, if compartments are crowded with muscles of large girth, or if postinjury fibrosis is present.

The IOM is then opened again with a long clamp and the excursion of the PTT is observed to ensure ease of passage and a course that is as straight as possible.

Several points must be considered at this time. First, is the PTT long enough to reach the proposed point of midfoot insertion? Second, is an isolated gastrocnemius recession or formal tendo-Achilles lengthening necessary? Third, are there residual medial soft-tissue contractures that need release or lengthening (eg, FHL, FDL, abductor hallucis, tarsal tunnel, plantar fascia, anterior deltoid, or hindfoot joint capsules)? These factors must be carefully addressed preoperatively and again intraoperatively.

When addressing medial contractures, the FHL and FDL tendons can be addressed by Z-lengthening, or a proximal recession performed at the musculotendinous junction. Release of the abductor hallucis often requires a circumferential fascial release along with release of the abductor-calcaneal fascial band, and even release of the abductor from its origin on the calcaneus. Plantar fascia release is usually adequate when 50% of the medial plantar fascia is transected. The authors prefer open releases with complete visualization of the small sensory and motor branches of the medial calcaneal and posterior tibial nerves, respectively. A complete tarsal tunnel release (including deep posterior crural fascia) may be necessary in severe long-standing equinovarus. Wound closure also becomes a concern in severe deformity, in which case an open in situ tarsal tunnel release may be performed, followed by gradual correction with a hinged circular fixator. The lead author does not advocate limited open or endoscopic tarsal tunnel releases as described by others[5] in severe deformity correction.

In cases with coexisting ankle varus, release of the superficial anterior deltoid ligament by "peeling" away the ligament from the bony attachments (much like medial ligamentous balancing in knee arthroplasty) is performed until the talus sits level (to within 5°) under the tibial plafond. If further medial ankle soft-tissue release is required, the surgeon should consider sequential release of the medial malleolar soft-tissue sleeve, the fibroosseous tunnels of the PT/FDL, the posteromedial joint capsule and ligamentous expansions, and finally the FDL/FHL sheaths and tendons.

Laterally, if adequate soft tissue structures are available, the ankle is stabilized with anatomic reconstructions; however, the lead author has found in most instances there is a paucity of available lateral tissue for an anatomic reconstruction. Thus, a nonanatomic reconstruction by means of a translateral malleolar peroneal tendon stabilization is required (ie, Broström-Evans). Supplemental reinforcement may be performed by any number of various modifications of periosteal turn-down[6] or ligament reefing procedures. After completing these very important ancillary releases and reconstructions, the final position and length of the PTT in relation to its new proposed insertion is reassessed. If the tendon length is adequate (PTT long enough to allow 25 mm of tunnel insertion), transfer is commenced.

Once any necessary medial contractures have been addressed, the PTT is next tunneled under the skin either with a tunneling tool or a long clamp. The tendon is passed and retrieved from the distal end. It is run back and forth to ensure appropriate gliding and to further create an adequate corridor for the tendon. The lead author prefer subcutaneous positioning because transferring the PTT under the inferior extensor retinaculum diminishes tendon length and power. If severe bow-stringing is a concern, reconstruction of the extensor retinaculum (both inferior and superior) with allograft material may be performed.[7]

If tendon length is inadequate, the surgeon may consider either a split turndown of the PTT (only if the PTT is of a robust caliber), a tendon graft (native peroneus tertius, peroneus brevis, or banked tendon allograft), or conversion to a bridle-type procedure (see later discussion). Typically, the tendon is inserted to the lateral cuneiform. Insertion may be achieved using a bony tunnel and an interference screw. In very muscular or large patients, patients with osteopenic bone, or patients with questionable ability to follow postoperative weight-bearing protocols, the authors recommend supplemental suture fixation to the osteo-periosteal tissues. In the authors' practice, supplemental fixation of traditional transosseous tendon placement with a skin bolster technique is still preferred over stand-alone interference screw fixation. To create such bolster fixation, a transosseous tunnel is created via serial drilling, ending with a final drill that best matches the caliber of the last 3 cm end of the transferred tendon. A long tag-stitch passed through the plantar skin with Keith needles and secured by suturing over a bolster or "button." Alternatively, the end of the suture tag may be sewn directly over the plantar fascia via a separate skin incision.[8]

The transferred tendon is tensioned with the ankle in neutral or slight (5°) of dorsiflexion. Temporary ankle/foot positioning may be accomplished by intraoperative pinning in the desired position with Kirschner wires, which may be removed at the end of the case, or at 2 to 4 weeks postoperatively (which is helpful in patients with spasticity, myoclonus, or dysarthritic neurologic disorders such as Parkinson disease).

Finally, articular stability of the foot and ankle is assessed, and any ligamentous balancing, bony stabilization (eg, arthrodeses), or osteotomies are performed. The first author has also performed simultaneous total ankle replacement with a posterior interosseous tendon transfer, placing the total ankle replacement first, followed by tendon transfers.[9]

In order to correct residual deformity after PTT transfer, on occasion, the lead author has found the need for ancillary soft tissue deformity correction with a small wire external fixator. The use of more traditional Ilizarov techniques or a spatial frame system becomes particularly germane and well-suited to tendon transfers when tibial realignments are required for bony deformity, such as malunions. Typically, the need for the spatial frame system may be assessed preoperatively through the physical examination and screening radiographs. In these complex cases a combined correction may be performed in closely spaced staged procedures.

All wounds are closed in layers, with particular attention to hemostasis (the tourniquet is released prior to closure). Drains are used as necessary. In spastic patients with myoclonus and anxiety-prone patients, an absorbable subcuticular running suture technique is used. Otherwise, interrupted nylon or skin staples are used. The lead author makes it a practice to leave in drains that have been placed in confined, small closed spaces (such as the foot) until the drain output is less than 15 cm^3 per 8 hours.

Bridle procedure

The bridle procedure is an excellent technique to achieve a plantigrade foot with an even distribution of dorsiflexion power. The bridle technique, first described in publication by McCall and colleagues in 101 patients, reported a 74% success rate (the authors also credited Brand and Riordan for the inception of the procedure).[10] Simultaneously, Rodriguez[11] reported favorable results, solidifying the procedure's popularity as a valid surgical option for dropfoot and equinovarus deformity. This technique is covered in depth elsewhere in this issue. The technique is best suited for correction of an acquired equinovarus foot when there is complete loss of peroneal function involving both the anterior and lateral compartments of the leg.[12] The lead author has found tremendous usefulness in the bridle procedure, even in the face of equinovarus, provided that the varus deformity can be adequately corrected and the varus deforming force can be neutralized.

Briefly, general anesthesia with neuromuscular blockade is used. In the bridle procedure and its modifications, the posterior tibial tendon plus the FHL or FDL tendons[9] are harvested and transferred to the anterior leg, above the ankle. The transferred tendons are tenodesed to both the tibialis anterior tendon (which remains in situ under the extensor retinaculum) and the peroneus longus (PL) tendon, creating a tritendon tenodesis. The lead author has found that using the PL is easier, provides a longer segment of tendon absent from impingement from muscle belly, and less frequently suffers from tendon tears. However, when lateral ankle ligament reconstruction is required, the lead author uses either peroneus brevis (PB) or PL for transfer, the choice dictated by the tendon quality available to accomplish both goals of tendon transfer and lateral ankle ligament reconstruction.

The surgical approach for harvesting the PTT and routing it through the IOM is similar to that of isolated PTT transfer. When transfer of the FDL or FHL tendons is required to augment the PT tendon, ancillary distal foot incisions are made at the digital sulcus of the great toe,[13] and the plantar-medial midfoot (arch area), allowing a long segment of tendon for transfer (**Fig. 4**). The anterior ankle/leg incision is similar and should allow acceptance of a distal incoming peroneal tendon. The IOM is widened sufficiently for passage of posterior tendons.

The peroneal tendon (PB or PL) is then harvested through a proximal incision at the level of the musculotendinous junction. The chosen peroneal tendon is transected as far proximally as possible and tagged. The remaining nontransferred tendon is either tenodesed to the muscular aponeurosis of the transferred tendon's muscle belly or used for augmentative tendon graft or lateral ankle ligament reconstruction. Next, a distal incision is made at the level of the base of the fifth metatarsal. The peroneal tendon is withdrawn from the proximal to the distal incision, followed by anterior subcutaneous passage to the level of the tendons to the anterior distal ankle/leg. This maneuver is facilitated by a curved clamp or a standard hand tendon retriever. Next, the tibialis anterior is identified, and the tendon's insertion is kept intact. The tibialis anterior proximal musculotendinous junction is either left in situ or transected, with the proximal cut end tagged. The peroneal tendon and tibialis anterior tendons are tenodesed to the posterior tendons that were transferred through the IOM. This is accomplished by multiple side-to-side tenodeses, or by weaving the posterior tendon and peroneal tendon through the more robust tibialis anterior tendon. Weaving may be facilitated by the use of a Pulvertaft tendon weaver (**Fig. 5**). Weaved or side-to-side tenodesed tendons are secured to one another with multiple interrupted sutures, completing a tritendon tenodesis (**Fig. 6**), with the posterior to anterior transfer (PTT with or without FHL/FDL) acting as the "motor" for the medially inserted "rope" (tibialis anterior) and the laterally inserted rope (PB or PL), providing even medial-lateral

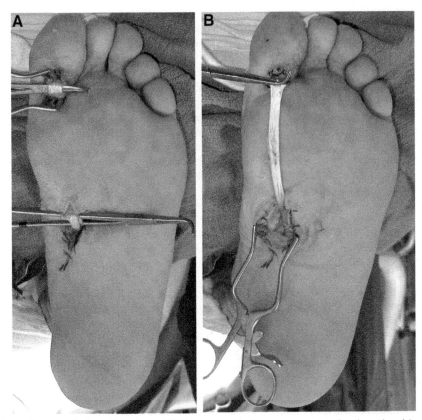

Fig. 4. (*A, B*) Technique for a long FHL harvest; note the generous tendon length achieved such that when transferred through the IOM, ample length is provided for any insertion point.

dorsiflexion tension when the posterior muscles contract. Barring poor suture technique,[14] it is the lead author's opinion that the integrity of tendon-suture interface is limited by the actual physical condition of the tendon (the tendon is the weakest link). Modern hybrid sutures (eg, Fiberwire, Arthrex, Naples, FL, USA) may cut through

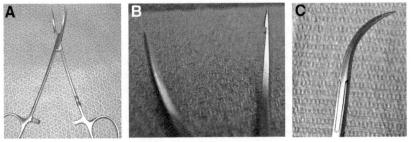

Fig. 5. Pulvertaft tendon weaver (*A*); note specialized tip designed for grasping donor tendon (*B*) and curved end (*C*) for weaving through recipient tendon.

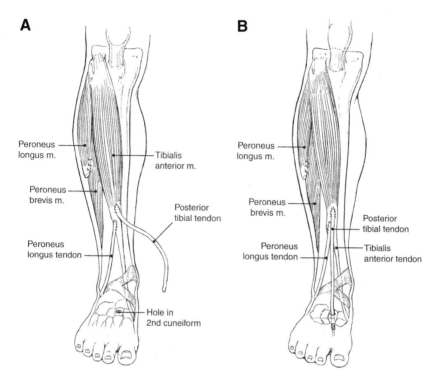

A

Peroneus longus m.

Tibialis anterior m.

Peroneus brevis m.

Posterior tibial tendon

Peroneus longus tendon

Hole in 2nd cuneiform

B

Peroneus longus m.

Peroneus brevis m.

Posterior tibial tendon

Peroneus longus tendon

Tibialis anterior tendon

Fig. 6. (*A, B*) The bridle tritendon anastomosis; remaining PTT may be inserted into the middle cuneiform, although frequently, sufficient length is not available to complete this maneuver. (*From* Myerson MS, editor. Foot & Ankle Disorders. Philadelphia (PA): WB Saunders; 2000. p. 888; with permission).

tendons. Because of this tendency, as well as a desire to minimize nonabsorbable foreign material, the authors prefer absorbable heavy sutures such as 0-0 or 2-0 Vicryl (Ethicon, Somerville, NJ, USA). To date, the authors have observed no adverse results (catastrophic or gradual tenodesis failure) from using absorbable suture material in tendon transfers.

Finally, after weaving and tenodesis of the PTT, if the length of harvested PTT is sufficient, it is inserted into the middle cuneiform as described for the isolated PTT transfer (see **Fig. 6**). A gastrocnemius-soleus complex release or Achilles lengthening is performed as needed based upon the intraoperative Silfverskiöld test. Ancillary medial soft tissue contractures are addressed (in the authors' experience these are usually less severe in patients selected for the bridle), along with tarsal tunnel release and lateral ankle ligament reconstruction as needed. Simultaneous arthrodesis, arthroplasty,[9] or osteotomies are executed.

Additional Posterior-to-Anterior Tendon Transfers for Equinovarus Deformity

Modifications of posterior-to-anterior tendon transfers have been reported. These techniques are valuable when there is weakness of a potential motor unit (eg, posterior tibialis) or physical loss of tendon structures (eg, absence of peroneal tendons from disease or trauma) and tendon transfer remains a viable option for return of function.

In 1980, Ono and colleagues[15] described their results after transfer of the FHL/FDL with equinus release for spastic equinovarus in 56 adults and children, yielding excellent results after 4-year follow-up. In 1994 Morita and colleagues[16] reported their results of that procedure pioneered by Ono.[15] In 1998, Morita and colleagues[17] reported their successful results in a larger series (n = 83) of patients who underwent FHL/FDL transfer combined with equinus release. The concept of transfer of the FHL/FDL for equinovarus (Ono-Morita procedure) is noteworthy, as it may be relatively unfamiliar to many surgeons. The lead author has adopted the concept of the Ono-Morita procedure in modifying the bridle procedure in a number of patients, with great success.

The patient is positioned supine and under general anesthesia as described previously. An extensile posteromedial incision allows identification and exposure of the FHL and FDL behind the ankle. The FHL is a more robust tendon and is preferentially used, with FDL supplementation as needed. The FHL is harvested distally past the master knot of Henry. In order to achieve maximum length of the harvested tendon, the Panchbhavi technique is recommended, in which the FHL is isolated in the midfoot, separated from the intertendinous attachments to the FDL, and then transected for harvest at the base of the great toe (see **Fig. 4**).[13] The FDL and FHL may be transferred singly or tenodesed as one unit and passed through a generous aperture in the IOM above the syndesmosis. The transferred tendons may be tenodesed to the anterior toe extensors/tibialis anterior, attached in bridle fashion or inserted into the cuneiforms. Secondary deforming forces (eg, PTT) are neutralized with fractional lengthening or split transfer. Secondarily contracted structures are also released.

Alternatively, transfer of the PTT to the tibialis anterior and then into the lateral cuneiform, combined with transfer of the FDL tendon to the extensor digitorum longus and extensor hallucis longus (EHL), has been described by Vigasio and colleagues.[18] When combined with appropriate releases, this procedure may be a viable alternative when isolated PTT transfer or the bridle procedure is not technically feasible. Wagenaar and colleagues[19] described the successful technique of a split PTT transfer through the IOM anastomosed only to the extensor tendons above the level of the ankle joint in young equinovarus patients. Mean dorsiflexion was to neutral but allowed ambulation without an ankle-foot orthosis (AFO) in over 90% of the patients in their series.

Split Tibialis Anterior Tendon Transfer for Equinovarus (Adult)

The split tibialis anterior transfer combined with an Achilles release has been a workhorse procedure for equinovarus since the 1960s.[20] It is discussed in detail in the pediatric section of this article. In adults, it has significant value when isolated tibialis anterior spasticity creates varus. The tibialis anterior is split and transferred to the lateral cuneiform. However, in a series of 125 patients with spastic equinovarus after CVA, Morita and colleagues[17] reported improved function and less recurrence of varus with FHL/FDL transfer compared with split tibialis anterior transfer, leading these investigators to abandon the use of the split tibialis anterior transfer for spastic equinovarus. As an alternative, equinovarus without tibialis anterior overactivity has been reported to be successfully treated by split EHL tendon transfer in combination with equinus release.[21]

Postoperative Care, Rehabilitation, and Expectations

Patients are typically admitted overnight, except for those with straightforward isolated PTT transfers who have undergone minimal ancillary procedures with excellent hemostasis. Admitted patients receive deep venous thrombosis prophylaxis with either fractionated heparin or unfractionated heparin (5000 units subcutaneous every 8 h). Postoperative pain control is facilitated by the use of patient-controlled analgesia pumps and peripheral indwelling pain catheters. When tarsal tunnel release has been performed, prophylactic gabapentin (600 mg 3 times daily) is prescribed. Transition to oral analgesics is routinely accomplished by the first postoperative day. Serial monitoring of wound healing, maintenance of foot position, and surveillance for deep venous thrombosis are critical, with a low threshold for ultrasound investigation of suspected thrombosis. Sutures are removed when the incision are healed and stabilized (approximately 4 week).

Patients are immobilized for 4 to 12 weeks postoperatively, depending on the quality of tendon fixation and ancillary procedure postoperative requirements. Generally, for the first 4 to 6 weeks they are kept nonweight bearing, followed by progression to full weight bearing at 8 weeks in cast or boot. By the 12th postoperative week, the lead author allows full unrestricted weight bearing in an AFO, and initiates formal tendon gliding as well as retraining and strengthening of the transferred muscle group in physical therapy. At this point in the postoperative period, ancillary releases are stable, osteotomies and fusions healed. An AFO is continued for 3 to 6 months, based on progression in rehabilitation. A rocker sole may be added to the patient's daily shoes, and heels are avoided. The previous are guidelines, and postoperative rehabilitation may be advanced based on individual patient assessments. For example, with simple releases and isolated tendon-tendon transfers in healthy, reliable patients, early active motion may be initiated as soon as 1 to 2 weeks postoperatively.[22]

The patient who undergoes a posterior-to-anterior tendon transfer for equinovarus deformity should be educated preoperatively about the goals of the surgery: to allow adequate foot clearance for gait or to allow the patient to wear an appropriate brace. In patients with more functional expectations, it should be stressed that the trade-off that occurs with these tendon transfers may be a limitation of plantarflexion motion. Additionally, full ankle dorsiflexion is usually not achieved, and dorsiflexion power does not match the contralateral limb. On occasion, in patients with severe weakness or those requiring multiple posterior-to-anterior transfers, the acceptable reality and outcome may be a functional tenodesis rather than an active motor transfer. In these patients as well as patients with continued spasticity from CVA or TBI, lifelong AFO bracing is recommended after tendon transfer.

TENDON TRANSFERS AND SURGICAL MANAGEMENT OF EQUINOVARUS DEFORMITIES IN CHILDREN AND ADOLESCENTS

The most common etiologies leading to an equinovarus deformity in young children and adolescents include

- Clubfoot deformity
- Equinovarus deformity due to spastic cerebral palsy
- Deformities due to imbalance of musculature secondary to neuropathic conditions such as spina bifida and progressive disease such as Charcot-Marie-Tooth disease
- Posttraumatic brain injuries from the brain leading to a muscular imbalance of the foot
- Rare congenital anomalies that lead to more rigid equinovarus deformities such as arthrogryposis.

The treatment of an equinovarus deformity depends on several factors. These include the underlying cause of the condition and the relative flexibility of the deformity during static examination. The particular imbalance that is generating the deformity must be considered in order to determine the appropriate tendon transfers. As with adults, the presence of soft-tissue contractures (including joint capsules) must be ascertained and may necessitate concomitant soft-tissue releases and hindfoot osteotomies.

The two most common tendon transfers used for correcting or balancing a pediatric equinovarus deformity of the foot are split anterior tibial tendon transfer (SPLATT) to the dorsum of the foot and split or complete posterior tibialis tendon transfer to the lateral aspect of the foot, usually suturing it into the peroneus brevis.

These transfers may be performed individually or occasionally combined. There have been various descriptions of where the tendon should be transferred or attached, including the classic Garceau transfer of the anterior tibialis to the peroneus brevis tendon to the lateral aspect of the foot.[23] More recently the transfer of the anterior tibialis to the dorsal midfoot has been adapted, to either the middle or lateral cuneiform bones, usually transferring the tendon into a bone tunnel.

The posterior tibialis tendon is traditionally transferred posterior to the tibia and the fibula and tenodesed to the peroneus brevis tendon. The tendon transfers are usually performed in conjunction with some soft tissue release as well, whether a tendo-Achilles lengthening, a gastrocnemius-soleus release, and/or release of hindfoot joint contractures.

Technique for Split Posterior Tibial Tendon Transfer (Garceau technique)

The patient is usually in the supine position. The incision begins at the navicular and curves around the medial malleolus. The posterior tibialis tendon is identified including its insertion into the navicular and the plantar aspect of the foot (**Fig. 7**A). The distal portion of the tendon sheath is exposed. The tendon is then split in half longitudinally and half is detached from its insertion near the plantar aspect of the navicular. Enough length should be maintained for transfer to the lateral foot. The end of the tendon is contoured so that it is not bulbous. The split half of the tendon is gradually teased and split to just behind the medial malleolus (see **Fig. 7**B). A section of the tendon sheath should be left intact. A second opening in the tendon sheath is made proximally and the split half of the tendon delivered under the malleolus and to the proximal aspect. The split is propagated to the musculotendinous junction. The nontransferred half of the tendon should remain attached to the navicular in its sheath.

The transferred portion is then transferred posteriorly behind the tibia and the fibula such that the tendon exits near the sheath of the peroneus brevis. A curved clamp is passed behind the tibia and the fibula from the medial incision until it exits in the subcutaneous tissue near the peroneal tendon sheath. A second incision is made in the lateral aspect of the foot just distal to the fibula at the level of the peroneal tendons. The peroneal tendon sheaths are opened and each tendon exposed and accurately identified. A curved tendon passer is now passed from the lateral wound to the medial wound, and the split posterior tibial tendon is then delivered to the lateral aspect of the ankle and tenodesed to the peroneus brevis tendon (see **Fig. 7**C). The tenodesis should be performed with the foot and ankle in neutral position and slight eversion. The tenodesis may be performed using a Pulvertaft weave, side-to-side anastomosis, or suture of the tendon directly through a split incision in the peroneus brevis. Once the tendon is transferred, the wounds are irrigated and closed in layers. The ankle should be immobilized in a posterior short-leg plaster splint or split short-leg cast.

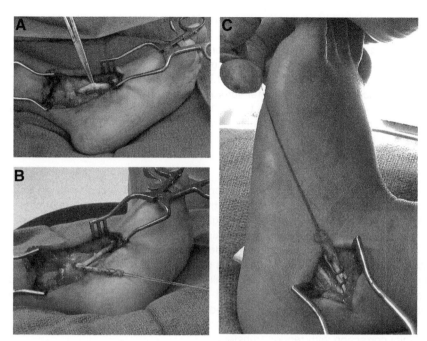

Fig. 7. (*A*) Incision, identification, and isolation of PTT. (*B*) Harvest and splitting of the PTT; tendon is tubularized, tagged, then routed posteriorly (see text). (*C*) Posteriorly transferred split PTT retrieved into a lateral incision over the peroneal tendons; the split PTT is anastomosed to the peroneus brevis tendo.

Technique for Transferring the Anterior Tibialis Tendon

Transfer of either the entire anterior tibialis or a portion of it (split anterior tibial tendon transfer) may be performed. The first incision allows harvest of the tendon from its insertion at the base of the cuneiform and first metatarsal. An oblique incision is made in the line of the tendon, and it is confirmed that the EHL is not mistaken for the tibialis anterior tendon. The latter has a broad insertion over the base of the cuneiform and first metatarsal. This can be peeled away entirely if the entire tendon is to be transferred, or the tendon can be split in half to transfer only the lateral half of the tendon. The tendon is detached from its insertion, sutured with a permanent suture, and tubularized. The septae of the tendon are then dissected subcutaneously proximally so that the tendon can be adequately mobilized. A second incision is then made in the distal portion of the anterior leg. The anterior tibialis tendon sheath is identified and opened. The transferred portion of the tendon is grasped and delivered into the anterior wound.

The transfer of the tendon is usually to the mid dorsum of the foot between the middle and lateral cuneiform. Whereas it can be transferred all the way to the peroneal tendon sheath, the authors' preference is to transfer the tendon to the dorsum of the foot between the cuneiforms. This location can be identified with fluoroscopy. A longitudinal incision is made over the dorsum of the foot between the middle and lateral cuneiform. The extensor brevis is dissected off in a subperiosteal manner.

There are multiple ways to secure the tendon including sutures, interference screws, and endo buttons. The authors' preference is to use a curved bony tunnel created by drilling one hole in the middle cuneiform, another in the lateral cuneiform, and then connecting the two with curettes. The drill holes should be large enough to accept the size of the anterior tibialis tendon to be transferred. The tendon is passed to the dorsum of the foot and passed through the tunnel. The tendon is usually pulled back and sutured upon itself with the foot in neutral dorsiflexed position with slight eversion if necessary. Supplemental sutures are also placed within the periosteum with permanent nonabsorbable material. Once the tendon is secured, wounds are irrigated and closed in layers. The ankle is immobilized in neutral or slight dorsiflexion using either a plaster splint or a split short-leg cast.

Complications

Complications to be considered are postoperative infection, wound healing issues, neurovascular injury, failure of the tendon transfer, and recurrence of deformity.

Wound infections usually consist of marginal areas of delayed healing and may be treated with local care. Concern should exist if wound healing problems occur over the anterior ankle/leg and transferred tendons. Preservation of the peroneus tertius muscle belly, which is usually low-lying, is prudent because simple transposition of the muscle belly to an area of poor skin healing may facilitate delayed primary closure or granulation of the site. Major wound sloughs are unusual and may require subatmospheric wound dressings, delayed skin grafting, or local fasciocutaneous flaps. Free tissue transfers are rarely required for wound coverage after equinovarus deformity correction with tendon transfers.

A more common wound problem is difficulty closing medial incisions after release of severe varus deformities. In these instances the choice may be made to place an immediate subatmospheric wound dressing with a delayed closure or close the incision in the deformed position and allow a gradual correction with an Ilizarov or small-wire spatial frame. In patients in whom limiting operative settings are desired and the support required for fine-wire corrections is prohibitive (eg, medical, health support, and cognitive reasons), the use of local flaps such as the abductor hallucis muscle flap may allow for simultaneous medial and plantar medial soft-tissue structure release and provide wound coverage.

Infection typically occurs in the setting of wound healing issues. The surgeon should be aggressive and not delay irrigation and debridement to facilitate local infection control, wound healing, and salvage of the tendon transfer. Antibiotic selection is based on deep operative cultures.

Failure of the tendon transfer, either gradual or catastrophic, may be treated with revision of the procedure, with close attention paid to the reasons why the tendon transfer failed. Possible contributing factors include incorrect indication, poor technique, materials failure, and patient noncompliance. Catastrophic failure may be more easily revised if failure occurs at the point of tendon insertion or tenodesis. Failure of the muscle-tendon unit of the motor may not be as easily salvaged; an attempt at a second transfer using the FDL/FHL may be attempted, provided these muscle-tendon units have not been previously included in the original transfer. Nonsalvageable failure of the tendon transfer may be best remedied with a tenodesis of the tibialis anterior and long-toe extensors to the anterior distal tibia ("stirrup" procedure) or arthrodesis. Recurrence of deformity, if detected early, may be mild and necessitate only additional releases of deforming forces and secondarily contracted structures. Consideration should be given to joint arthrodesis (eg, transverse tarsal, subtalar joints) to supplement mild to moderate deformity recurrence. Severe recurrence of deformity may be recalcitrant to revision soft-tissue surgery alone, and more often than not requires multiple fusions of the foot and ankle to maintain a plantigrade foot position.

When a subretinacular path is chosen for tendon transfer, acute dynamic vascular compromise may occur. If recognized intraoperatively, the tendon should be rerouted subcutaneously. If recognized late, the foot should be carefully assessed for the need for rerouting of the transferred tendon. Acute arterial vascular injury should be repaired in the standard fashion; however, chronically shorted vessels (eg, posterior tibial artery injury) may require vein grafting.

Neurologic complications may occur acutely or late and include a range of complications from paresthesias to frank anesthesia (nerve transection), neuroma formation, and complex regional pain syndromes (CRPS). Paresthesias are treated expectantly and allowed up to 18 months to resolve. CRPS is treated immediately with pharmacologic therapy, physical therapy (desensitization, edema control, and range of motion when appropriate), and sympathetic blockade. Nerve transection should be suspected if there is a dense paresthesia that does not show improvement over a short course of time (2 wk) and is supported by electrodiagnostic testing. End-to-end repair is performed, but if this is not possible, nerve conduits should be placed. Neuroma formation is uncommon and should be treated stepwise with recalcitrant cases requiring neuroma resection and nerve reconstruction. More typical is the discovery of either an acute or evolving compressive neuropathy in the distribution of the posterior tibial nerve and its terminal branches that occurs after deformity correction. Expedient release of the tarsal tunnel should be performed. This complication may be prevented by performing a prophylactic tarsal tunnel release.

SUMMARY

Tendon transfers for the equinovarus foot in the adult and pediatric population continue to enjoy high success rates for correction of deformity and improvements in ambulation that translate to an improved quality of life. A host of tendon transfer options exist when standard techniques are unable to be used. The recent addition of the Ilizarov technique and spatial small-wire frame for gradual corrections adds an enhanced element in the correction of severe deformity.

ACKNOWLEDGMENTS

The lead author and Elsevier wish to acknowledge the wonderful secretarial assistance of Susan "Grammy" Nilsen of Mexico Beach, Florida.

REFERENCES

1. Carda S, Bertoni M, Zerbinati P, et al. Gait changes after tendon functional surgery for equinovarus foot in patients with stroke: assessment of temporo-spatial, kinetic, and kinematic parameters in 177 patients. Am J Phys Med Rehabil 2009;88(4):292–301.
2. Garozzo D, Ferraresi S, Buffatti P. Surgical treatment of common peroneal nerve injuries: indications and results. A series of 62 cases. J Neurosurg Sci 2004;48(3): 105–12 [discussion: 112].
3. Watkins MB, Jones JB, Ryder CJ, et al. Transplantation of the posterior tibial tendon. J Bone Joint Surg [Am] 1954;36:1181–9.
4. Bibbo C, Patel DV, Gehrmann RM, et al. Chlorhexidine provides superior skin decontamination in foot and ankle surgery: a prospective randomized study. Clin Orthop Relat Res 2005;438:204–8.
5. Day FN 3rd, Naples JJ. Endoscopic tarsal tunnel release: update 96. J Foot Ankle Surg 1996;35(3):225–9.

6. Tan VK, Lin SS, Okereke E. Superior peroneal retinaculoplasty: a surgical technique for peroneal subluxation. Clin Orthop Relat Res 2003;(410):320–5.

7. Bibbo C. The small intestinal submucosa (SIS) patch in reconstructive foot & ankle surgery. J Foot Ankle Surg 2010;49:123–7.

8. Bibbo C, Anderson RB, Davis WH, et al. Repair of Achilles tendon sleeve avulsions: quantitative and functional evaluation of transcalcaneal suture technique. Foot Ankle Int 2003;24:539–44.

9. Bibbo C, Baronofsky HJ, Jaffe L. Combined total ankle replacement and modified bridle tendon transfer for end-stage ankle joint arthrosis with paralytic dropfoot: report of an unusual case. J Foot Ankle Surg 2011;50:453–7.

10. McCall RE, Frederick HA, McCluskey GM, et al. The Bridle procedure: a new treatment for equinus and equinovarus deformities in children. J Pediatr Orthop 1991;11(1):83–9.

11. Rodriguez RP. The Bridle procedure in the treatment of paralysis of the foot. Foot Ankle 1992;13:63–9.

12. Steinau HU, Tofaute A, Huellmann K, et al. Tendon transfers for drop foot correction: long-term results including quality of life assessment, and dynamometric and pedobarographic measurements. Arch Orthop Trauma Surg 2011;131(7):903–10.

13. Panchbhavi VK. Chronic Achilles tendon repair with flexor hallucis longus tendon harvested using a minimally invasive technique. Techniques in Foot and Ankle Surgery 2007;6(2):123–9.

14. Bibbo C, Milia M, Gehrmann, RM, et al. Strength and knot security of braided polyester and caprolactone/glycolide suture. Foot Ankle Int 2004;25:712–5.

15. Ono K, Hiroshima K, Tada K, et al. Anterior transfer of the toe flexors for equinovarus deformity of the foot. Int Orthop 1980;4(3):225–9.

16. Morita S, Yamamoto H, Furuya K. Anterior transfer of the toe flexors for equinovarus deformity due to hemiplegia. J Bone Joint Surg [Br] 1994;76(3):447–9.

17. Morita S, Muneta T, Yamamoto H, et al. Tendon transfer for equinovarus deformed foot caused by cerebrovascular disease. Clin Orthop Relat Res 1998;(350):166–73.

18. Vigasio A, Marcoccio I, Patelli A, et al. New tendon transfer for correction of drop-foot in common peroneal nerve palsy. Clin Orthop Relat Res 2008;466(6):1454–66.

19. Wagenaar FC, Louwerens JW. Posterior tibial tendon transfer: results of fixation to the dorsiflexors proximal to the ankle joint. Foot Ankle Int 2007;28:1128–42.

20. Mooney V, Goodman F. Surgical approaches to lower-extremity disability secondary to strokes. Clin Orthop Relat Res 1969;63:142–52.

21. Carda S, Molteni F, Bertoni M, et al. Extensor hallucis longus transfer as an alternative to split transfer of the tibialis anterior tendon to correct equinovarus foot in hemiplegic patients without overactivity of tibialis anterior. J Bone Joint Surg [Br] 2010;92(9):1262–6.

22. Rath S, Schreuders TA, Stam HJ, et al. Early active motion versus immobilization after tendon transfer for foot drop deformity: a randomized clinical trial. Clin Orthop Relat Res 2010;468(9):2477–84.

23. Garceau GJ. Talipesequino-varus. Instr Course Lect 1955;12:90–9.

The Bridle Procedure

David R. Richardson, MD*, L. Nathan Gause, MD

KEYWORDS

- Bridle procedure • Drop-foot • Cerebral palsy • Leprosy
- Traumatic brain injury • Peroneal nerve palsy

The "bridle" procedure is a modification of the transfer of the tibialis posterior to the dorsum of the foot for the treatment of a supple equinus or equinovarus deformity of the ankle and hindfoot.[1–4] It consists of a transfer of the posterior tibial tendon through the interosseous membrane to the dorsum of the foot with concomitant anastomosis to the anterior tibial and peroneus longus tendons. It is indicated primarily in the setting of a drop-foot and a steppage gait, which is awkward, energy consuming, and physically limiting.[3,5] In affected patients, even a partial correction of this gait pattern may decrease or eliminate the need for bracing. This can be of great benefit, especially if other disabilities accompany the loss of ankle dorsiflexion. In patients who have even limited lower or upper neuron pathology, lack of dorsiflexion of the foot can markedly change function and lifestyle.

HISTORY

Transfer of the tibialis posterior muscle–tendon unit to the dorsum of the foot, either around the medial malleolus or through the interosseous membrane, has been used for the treatment of drop-foot deformity for over half a century, with many retrospective reviews documenting its utility.[6–13] The genesis of the bridle modification of a well-documented muscle–tendon motor unit[3] transposition (bony insertion to bony insertion) or transfer (tendon to tendon) is unclear, but it generally is credited to Dr Daniel Riordan.[2] However, the modification of the standard single transfer of the tibialis posterior tendon in the treatment of drop-foot deformity in patients with leprosy may have its origins with Dr Paul Brand at the Christian Medical College of Valore, India. Dr Brand performed groundbreaking research on the upper and lower extremity neural damage afflicting patients with leprosy, including both motor and sensory loss. The common peroneal nerve at the neck of the fibula, the posterior tibial nerve within the tarsal tunnel, and the ulnar nerve at the medial epicondyle of the elbow are frequent targets of the *Mycobacterium leprae* organism. While in India, where bracing is difficult to effect and maintain,

Campbell Clinic Foundation, University of Tennessee-Campbell Clinic, 1211 Union Avenue, Memphis, TN 38104, USA
* Corresponding author.
E-mail address: drrichardson@campbellclinic.com

Foot Ankle Clin N Am 16 (2011) 419–433
doi:10.1016/j.fcl.2011.06.003
1083-7515/11/$ – see front matter © 2011 Elsevier Inc. All rights reserved.

Selvapandian and Brand described transfer of the tibialis posterior to the dorsum of the foot.[9]

When Brand became Director of the Leprosorium at Carville, Louisiana, he and a noted hand surgeon, Dr Daniel C. Riordan of New Orleans, collaborated on studies of the complexities of the anatomy and physiology of skeletal muscle. In addition, they investigated the biomechanics and surgical techniques of a number of muscle–tendon unit transfers and transpositions in patients with leprosy. Dr Riordan had extensive experience with tendon transfers in combat injuries of the upper and lower extremities in the immediate aftermath of World War II, and both surgeons had wide experience with the myriad combinations of muscle function loss in poliomyelitis. Dr Riordan for many years consulted and taught at the Shriners Hospital for Crippled Children in Shreveport, Louisiana, where he extended this knowledge to patients with spasticity and drop-foot deformity. It was out of these circumstances that the bridle procedure was born. Later, patients with drop-foot secondary to hereditary motor sensory neuropathies, as well neurologic impairments from upper and lower central motor neuron injury and diseases, were considered candidates for this procedure. Its purpose was to aid in the balance of the multiplanar deformity of the foot and ankle—equinus of the ankle and varus and supination of the foot.[2,4]

Why was the bridle procedure conceived? A number of publications in peer-reviewed journals confirmed and even extolled the merits of the standard technique of transferring the tibialis posterior through the interosseous membrane or around the medial aspect of the distal tibia in selected patients with a broad spectrum of diagnoses.[2,3,10,13] There are 5 reasons to alter the technique of transferring the tibialis posterior to the dorsum of the foot surfaced after various institutions reported complications of both the interosseous or perimalleolar technique.

1. Troublesome sequelae (recurrence of deformity and instability of the hindfoot) with the technique of subcutaneously routing the tibialis posterior to the dorsum of the foot were reported.[6,8]
2. Including the peroneus longus and tibialis anterior tendons as a combined tendon "junctura" was considered more likely to secure a "balanced foot and ankle" when treating a multiplanar deformity (equinus, varus and supination) resulting from a "high" peroneal nerve injury where both the anterior and lateral compartment musculature were lost.[4,5]
3. This multiple tendon weave also was an attempt at balancing the foot in a spastic patient population where multiplanar deformity is the rule and in whom balance is difficult to maintain, not only in the foot and ankle, but also in the body as a whole.[2]
4. By suturing the "junctura" of tendons greater than or equal to 2 cm proximal to the superior peroneal retinaculum, maximal excursion of the transferred motor tendon unit was possible without abutment on the extensor pulley.[14]
5. Suturing the transfer to the tibialis anterior and peroneus longus tendons eliminated the need for a bony tunnel and the problem of determining the maximally beneficial location for tendon insertion in the dorsal midfoot.[3,4]

However, reports that this bridle modification stretched out over a prolonged period of time with recurrence of the deformity and instability of the hindfoot and midfoot led to yet another modification to this transfer.[5] It was Dr Raoul Rodriguez who proposed the current technique to prevent elongation of the transfer and recurrent deformity. This modification of the original procedure combines bony insertion of the tibialis posterior into the center of the midfoot (middle cuneiform) with the customary tri-tendon weave (tibialis posterior, tibialis anterior, and peroneus longus) in the distal anterior leg.[4,7]

This technique of securing the transferred, centrally placed motor–tendon unit into bone while rebalancing a supple multiplanar deformity by combining an inverter (tibialis anterior) and everter (peroneus longus) muscle–tendon unit to the central stabilizing transfer was adopted in an attempt to improve the predictability of surgical correction. Whether it would prevent recurrence in patients with spasticity and particularly those with severe spastic quadriplegia/diplegia was uncertain; however, this modification of the bridle procedure was reported to improve the beneficial results of the original procedure: Long-term balance of the foot and ankle that eliminated or reduced the need for brace use, improved gait, and reduced shoe wear concerns.

ADVANTAGES

Uniplanar and multiplanar (equinus and equinovarus) deformities of the foot and ankle (drop-foot deformity) are treatable with the bridle procedure.[2,4,9,12–14] Deformities with multiple etiologies can be treated as well, including peripheral nerve injury (common peroneal nerve loss affecting both eversion and dorsiflexion of the foot and ankle or deep peroneal nerve loss affecting dorsiflexion).[4–6] Active function of the transfer is predictable with this diagnosis. With an L5 nerve root deficit, the transfer not only corrects the drop-foot deformity, but also provides a degree of active function of the transfer.[4,5] The bridle procedure is a good choice in spastic paralysis from upper motor neuron injury at the cord or motor cortex level because voluntary control of the transfer(s) in this setting is unpredictable.[2,4,8,11,13] Leprosy remains a formidable challenge to orthopaedic surgeons in some parts of the world. These patients may benefit greatly, even though sensory deficits can lead to complications that are unlikely in the sensate foot.[9,10] Patients with lumbar myelodysplasia and spinal dysraphism, as well as Friedrich's ataxia and muscular dystrophy, most often are under the care of a pediatric orthopaedic surgeon and neurologist; however, the bridle procedure may be of benefit in very carefully selected patients.[2,13]

Even though transfers in compartment syndrome with loss of the anterior and/or lateral compartments of the leg frequently function only as a tenodesis, the dorsiflexed position is of benefit to the patient.[3,5,12] Results of transfer for drop-foot deformity caused by hereditary motor and sensory neuropathies (eg, Charcot–Marie–Tooth disease) are unpredictable. Because of the progressive nature, a hindfoot stabilization procedure (eg, triple arthrodesis) should be considered before the transfer to increase the probability of maintaining long-term correction.[2,13]

The modification of the bridle procedure described by Rodriguez allows predictable satisfactory long-term results even if the transfer functions solely as a tenodesis, as do many of the isolated tibialis posterior transfers for drop-foot.[3,4]

DISADVANTAGES

The bridle procedure is technically demanding. Multiple incisions are required, particularly if multiplanar deformities—dorsiflexion and eversion—are corrected. Setting the tension of 2 transferred motor tendon units (tibialis anterior and posterior) and 1 static tendon (peroneus longus) is challenging. There is the potential for loss of excursion of the transposed tibialis posterior tendon at the interosseous membrane window because of fibrosis. The superficial peroneal nerve, if it is spared in a uniplanar drop-foot deformity, may be injured (deep peroneal nerve injury only). There is potential for the development of a calcaneus deformity when combined with a heel cord lengthening, particularly in patients with spasticity or myelodysplasia.[4,6,9,11] A palpable and visible mass in the distal anterior compartment is possible, especially if the transfer is superficial to the superior extensor retinaculum.

Outcomes in spastic paralysis (cerebral palsy, traumatic closed head injury, cerebrovascular accident) are unpredictable with the bridle procedure.[8,11] Other than leprosy and cerebral palsy, most studies include multiple etiologies for the motor deficit(s). Wide variations in age and comorbidities are seldom considered.[5,6,11] Except for patients with diagnoses of cerebral palsy or leprosy, the number of patients in any given study are limited.[4,6]

CLINICAL OUTCOMES

Transfer of the tibialis posterior through the interosseous membrane for drop-foot deformity has been widely studied in retrospective reviews of patients with a spectrum of diagnoses, ages, and settings; however, there are only a few retrospective studies published reporting the bridle procedure for the correction of drop-foot deformity.[2,4,5]

McCall and colleagues[2] reported the largest series, with 128 bridle procedures in 101 children, most of whom had spastic cerebral palsy. Better results (80% excellent/good) were obtained in children with hemiplegia than in those with diplegia (68% excellent/good). The risk of deformity recurrence was higher in those with severe involvement (diplegia and quadriplegia). Calcaneus deformities (in 13 feet) were the most serious complication in cerebral palsy patients; 6 of the 13 patients required further surgery. Because 12 of 13 calcaneus deformities developed in 6 patients who had severe bilateral lower limb spasticity, the authors recommended caution in using the bridle procedure in patients with severe spasticity.

Rodriguez[4] modified the bridle procedure by placing the tibialis posterior tendon into bone (middle cuneiform) rather than depending on the tri-tendon weave above the ankle to maintain dorsiflexion in 10 of 11 transfers in patients with varied etiologies for their deformities. He reported better results in patients with flaccid paralysis than in those with cerebral palsy.

In their review of 10 bridle procedures in 10 military patients, most of whom had traumatic peroneal nerve injury, Prahinski and colleagues[5] reported that the bridle procedure is beneficial for patients with low physical demands, but that it may stretch out over time and fail in patients with high demands. In this small group of patients, concurrent peroneal nerve exploration and repair did not seem to be beneficial.

Although the numbers of patients for whom the bridle procedure is indicated are small,[1,6,7] these 3 peer-reviewed publications indicate that it can be effective in both children and adults with a variety of etiologies for their drop-foot deformities. Given the concerns about late loss of dorsiflexion in patients with high physical demands,[5] the Rodriquez modification[7] seems to be appropriate. Although the exact benefits of the procedure over the standard transfer of the tibialis posterior through the interosseous membrane are not entirely clear, the bridle procedure does provide improved balance of the correction in patients with varying diagnoses resulting in foot-drop.

PREOPERATIVE CONSIDERATIONS

Patients with spasticity should be examined by a neurologist to confirm the type of underlying injury or disease. Athetosis, ataxia, and any other neurologic deficit, if unrecognized, could compromise the outcome. In patients with peroneal nerve injury, careful assessment of the lateral, anterior, and posterior compartment musculature as to strength and excursion is essential. A physiatrist and/or neurologist should perform an electromyelogram and nerve conduction velocity test of the entire lower extremity as well as the paraspinal muscles. In patients with peroneal nerve injury, a repeat electrical study and detailed physical examination with grading of the strength of the involved muscles should be done before surgery to be certain return of function is unlikely.

Generally, a 12- to 18-month period should lapse between injury and surgery in patients with peroneal nerve injury or compartment syndrome, although there are exceptions to this guidance. With segmental nerve loss, extensive débridement of 1 or more muscle compartments, or extenuating socioeconomic influences, combined with definitive objective findings on physical examination and electrical studies, the patient's interests may be best served by proceeding earlier with transfer.

The tibialis posterior muscle–tendon unit should have at least four fifths of its strength with nearly normal passive motion of the mid-foot–hind-foot complex. This implies normal or nearly normal excursion (2 cm) of the muscle–tendon unit transfer. A normal heel-to-toe gait with normal length of stance and swing phases of the gait cycle usually are not present after transfer, and the patient and family must be aware of this; however, marked improvement in 1 or more of the indications for the surgery should be expected. Although the goal is to allow the patient to be brace-free, for extended periods of exercise, bracing may be required even after a successful transfer and satisfactory functional result. Again, the patient and family must be aware of this before the procedure is performed.

Postoperative protection of the transfer is essential and the patient must be able to cooperate with and physically perform directives in the rehabilitation of the extremity. Any patient who has not given brace management of the drop-foot a concerted effort should be cautioned against having this extensive procedure, which is designed for functional and not cosmetic improvement.[2,4,5,7]

AUTHORS' INDICATIONS AND PREFERRED TECHNIQUE

Our most common indications for performing a bridle procedure include (1) posttraumatic common peroneal nerve deficit; (2) after debridement of the anterior compartment musculature; (3) Charcot-Marie-Tooth disease (hind-foot stabilization before transfer if patient has fixed hind-foot varus too severe to correct with calcaneal osteotomy); (4) spastic hemiplegia without fixed deformity; and (5) L5 nerve root deficit.

Concomitant lengthening of the Achilles is often necessary. For severe fixed ankle equinus, an open Z-lengthening is preferred. For ankle equinus correctable to −10°,

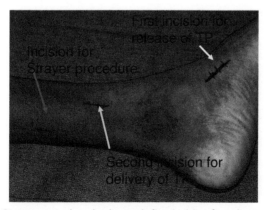

Fig. 1. Incision for Strayer procedure (*red arrow*), first incision for release of tibialis posterior (*yellow arrow*), second incision for proximal delivery of tibialis posterior (*green arrow*).

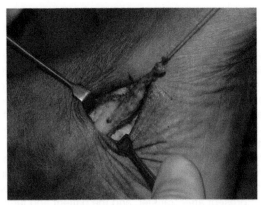

Fig. 2. Incision #1 may need to be lengthened if significant adhesions are present.

triple hemi-section (Hoke) will usually suffice. Finally, a Strayer gastrocnemius recession[15] is indicated in the setting of a gastrocnemius contracture (passive dorsiflexion to or past neutral with knee flexed). If trying to choose between a Strayer and Hoke procedure, the Strayer procedure is preferred because a calcaneus gait is not well tolerated. Caution is advised before performing an Achilles lengthening in conjunction with the bridle procedure in patients with spastic quadriplegia or diplegia, myelodysplasia, or muscular dystrophy.[6,4,10]

Operative Technique

After complete relaxation of the extremity with either general or regional anesthesia, a bolster is placed under the ipsilateral hip. A thigh tourniquet is used. Incision #1 is a 4 to 6 cm linear incision over the medial foot centered over the navicular tuberosity (**Fig. 1**). The slip of the tibialis posterior inserting on the navicular tuberosity is isolated. The anterior and posterior margins of this slip are determined and dissection is extended 1 to 2 cm distal to the tuberosity, raising the periosteum with the tendon.

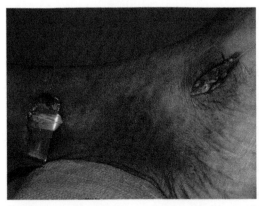

Fig. 3. Deliver the tibialis posterior into the proximal wound by applying traction to the tendon.

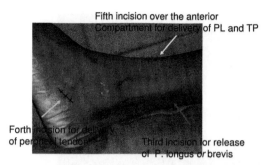

Fifth incision over the anterior
Compartment for delivery of PL and TP

Forth incision for delivery
of peroneal tendon

Third incision for release
of P. longus or brevis

Fig. 4. Incision #3 for release of the peroneus longus or brevis (*red arrow*), incision #4 for delivery of the peroneal tendon (*green arrow*), and incision #5 over the anterior compartment for delivery of the peroneal tendon and tibialis posterior.

Traction is placed on the tendon to give a sense of its excursion and if tethering may prevent retrieval in the proximal wound (**Fig. 2**).

Incision #2 is made in the distal leg along the tendon if it is palpable beneath the flexor digitorum longus tendon. In thin patients, the posteromedial tibial surface is palpated, whereas tension is placed on the distal end of the released tendon. If not palpable, the incision begins 1 to 2 cm distal to the junction of the middle third and distal third of the tibia and is extended proximally 4 to 6 cm to expose the musculotendinous junction by retracting the flexor digitorum longus posteriorly. The tendon is then delivered into the proximal wound (**Fig. 3**).

Incision #3 is made along the posterolateral border of the fibula, beginning 6 to 8 cm proximal to the tip of the fibula and extending 4 to 6 cm proximally to expose the musculotendinous junction of the peroneus longus (**Fig. 4**). The sural nerve should be posterior to the incision but its course is variable. The peroneus longus tendon is transected at its musculotendinous junction. The proximal end of the tendon is

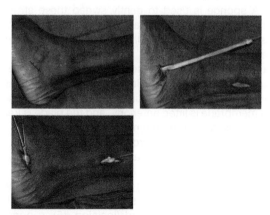

Fig. 5. The sural nerve is identified and protected. The peroneus longus tendon is identified as it courses toward the cuboid groove. The proximal end of the transected tendon is then delivered into the distal wound. If the peroneus brevis is of sufficient length, it provides greater eversion strength owing to its insertion of the base of the 5th metatarsal. In this patient, the peroneus longus was chosen.

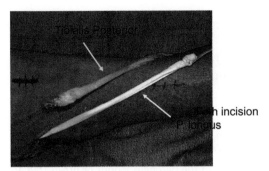

Fig. 6. Incision #5 (*red arrow*) is continued distally until it overlaps the posteromedial (second) incision by 1 cm. This allows a more direct course of the transferred peroneus longus tendon (*yellow arrow*).

pulled distally to maximal length, then relaxed until approximately 50% of its excursion is reached. At this tension, it is sutured to the peroneus brevis tendon. If the tendon of origin of the peroneus brevis is "teased" away from its muscle of origin and is found to be sufficient in length and substance, transferring the peroneus brevis tendon to the anterior compartment provides more eversion activity than transfer of the peroneus longus because of its insertion at the base of the 5th metatarsal.

Next, a 3- to 4-cm longitudinal incision (incision #4) is made at the inferior margin of the calcaneocuboid joint (see **Fig. 4**). The sural nerve is identified and protected. The peroneus longus tendon is identified as it courses toward the cuboid groove. The proximal end of the transected tendon is then delivered into the wound (**Fig. 5**).

Incision #5 is begun 2 cm lateral to the anterior border of the tibia and 4 to 6 cm proximal to the posteromedial incision. This incision is continued distally until it overlaps the posteromedial incision by 1 cm. This allows a more direct course of the transferred peroneus longus tendon (**Fig. 6**). The tibialis anterior, extensor digitorum longus, extensor hallucis longus, and peroneus tertius musculotendinous units are retracted laterally. A sponge is used to gently sweep these structures toward the fibula to expose the interosseous membrane throughout the length of the incision. Once the interosseous membrane is fully exposed, the adjacent neurovascular structures also are protected (**Fig. 7**).

A scalpel with a small, round edge is used to carefully penetrate the interosseous membrane. Incising along the posteromedial tibia allows the interosseous membrane to be lifted anteriorly as the release is continued distally. The released medial margin of the interosseous membrane is lifted anteriorly, and the blade is kept at a depth only sufficient to incise this thin structure from medial to lateral until the fibula is reached. If there was a previous compartment syndrome, the membrane may be thickened and more difficult to elevate. Once the fibular margin is reached, 5 to 6 cm of the interosseous membrane is excised.

At the posteromedial wound (incision #2) a suture is placed into the distal end of the tibialis posterior tendon (2-0 Fiberwire on a small needle with a Kessler grasping stitch is suggested). Through the anterior wound (incision #5), a periosteal elevator is gently inserted along the posterior border of the tibia, remaining next to bone until the instrument rests in the posteromedial wound. With this instrument as a guide, a small tendon passer or clamp is slid along the surface of this "guide" and into the medial wound (incision #2). The end of the suture is grasped and the tibialis

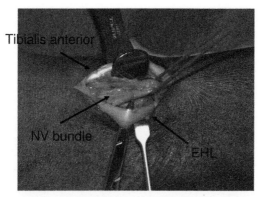

Fig. 7. The tibialis anterior, extensor digitorum longus, extensor hallucis longus, and peroneus tertius musculotendinous units are retracted (usually laterally) to expose the interosseous membrane throughout the length of the incision.

posterior is delivered into the anterior wound (incision #5). With a gentle pull on the muscle–tendon unit and finger dissection along its anterior, posterior, medial, and lateral margins, the tibialis posterior muscle is freed circumferentially until it has as straight a course as possible toward its intended insertion. Muscle rather than tendon should be visible in the interosseous membrane window. The ankle is dorsiflexed to neutral and maintained in that position. Proximal traction is then applied to the tibialis anterior tendon to hold the ankle in neutral dorsiflexion without assistance.

With the ankle in this position, a 2-cm longitudinal (sagittal plane) incision is made in the tibialis anterior tendon, 3 to 5 cm proximal to the superior extensor retinaculum. The tibialis posterior tendon is passed through this incision from posterior to anterior. With the ankle in 5 degrees of dorsiflexion and a firm pull placed on the tibialis posterior, the tendon is sutured to the tibialis anterior with a nonabsorbable suture.

From incision #5 in the anterior compartment, a tunnel is made from proximal to distal, superficial to the extensor retinaculum, to the lateral foot wound (incision #4).

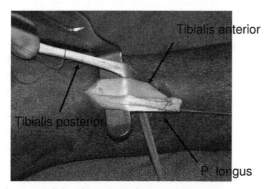

Fig. 8. All 3 tendons used in the tri-tendon anastomosis are now in the anterior compartment.

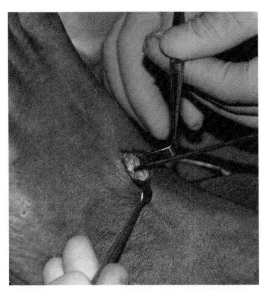

Fig. 9. The periosteum of the appropriate cuneiform (usually the intermediate or lateral) is incised and a guide pin is placed to prepare a tunnel through which the tibialis posterior tendon is to be passed.

A tendon passer is used to bring the peroneus longus tendon into the anterior compartment. All 3 tendons used in the tri-tendon anastomosis are now in the anterior compartment (**Fig. 8**).

Incision #6 is a 3-cm incision on the dorsum of the mid-tarsus 1 cm lateral to the dorsalis pedis artery. This is facilitated by marking the course of the artery before inflation of the tourniquet. The neurovascular bundle is identified and retracted medially. The cuneiform bones are identified, by image intensification if necessary. The periosteum of the appropriate cuneiform (usually the intermediate or lateral) is incised and a guide pin is placed to prepare a tunnel through which the tibialis posterior tendon is to be passed (**Fig. 9**). A biotenodesis screw set is preferred because it allows precise sizing of the tunnel to fit the tendon. The cuneiform bones are particularly small and placement as well as direction of the drilling must be precise (**Fig. 10**). The bony tunnel is created before delivery of the tibialis posterior into the dorsal foot wound (incision #6) so that the ankle can be plantarflexed without proximal migration of the tibialis posterior.

The tibialis posterior tendon is now identified in the anterior compartment wound (incision #5). It is subcutaneously tunneled from proximal to distal and passed superficial to the extensor retinaculum. This maximizes the power of the transfer yet results in "bowstringing," which should be discussed with the patient preoperatively.

The ends of the previously placed suture are grasped and used to gently bring the tibialis posterior tendon into the distal wound (incision #6; **Fig. 11**). The tendon is carefully trimmed while the suture weave is protected. The ends of the suture are placed through the eye of a straight needle, and the needle is passed through the prepared hole in the cuneiform, exiting the plantar aspect of the foot. Once both suture ends exit the foot plantarly, the suture is pulled distally while the tendon is guided into the bony tunnel and the ankle is held in 5 to 10 degrees of dorsiflexion. It is then secured in the tunnel.

The options for securing the tendon include an interference screw, suture anchor, or tying the suture ends over a plantar button which has been heavily padded with felt or gauze. Because secure fixation of the tibialis posterior is critical to the success of the procedure, we use all 3 fixation methods (**Figs. 12** and **13**). The tibialis posterior tendon should now hold the ankle at neutral or slightly dorsiflexed.

At the anterior wound (incision #3), the peroneus longus tendon is passed through the tibialis anterior tendon as follows: A #11 blade is used to incise the tibialis anterior from lateral to medial beginning at least 1 cm proximal to the opening through which the tibialis posterior was passed. The opening should be wide enough to allow the peroneus longus tendon to pass freely through the tendon. While the tibialis anterior tendon is pulled proximally, maintaining the dorsiflexed position of the ankle, sufficient tension is placed on the peroneus longus tendon (which has been placed through the tibialis anterior tendon) to evert the foot a few degrees. While appropriate tension is placed on the peroneus longus tendon, side-to-side sutures are placed to secure the tendon to the tibialis anterior. The tri-tendon weave is now complete (**Fig. 14**).

The end of the peroneus longus is brought proximally and sutured side to side to the tibialis anterior; any excess tendon is excised. This will plantar flex the first ray slightly. An additional optional stitch is suggested to reduce tension on the tri-tendon weave: A simple "box" stitch placed 1 cm proximal and 1 cm distal to the previous incisions in the tibialis anterior where the tibialis posterior and peroneus longus tendons pass. This "box stitch" should be under sufficient tension to produce a

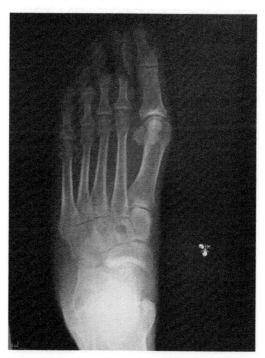

Fig. 10. The bone tunnel is placed most often in the intermediate or lateral cuneiform. Because of incomplete peroneal weakness, the intermediate cuneiform was chosen in this patient.

minimal "accordion affect" at the tendon weave to reduce tension on the multiple suture lines during initial healing.

With a bolster under the calf, the position in which the ankle is resting is inspected. There should be no equinus. The tourniquet is released, hemostasis is obtained, and the multiple wounds are closed in a nontensioned, everted fashion. Effort should be made to repair the fascia of the anterior compartment to minimize the soft-tissue mass on the anterior leg resulting from the tri-tendon weave (**Fig. 15**).

POSTOPERATIVE CARE

A bulky, conforming, soft dressing is applied followed by posterior and stirrup plaster splints. At 12 to 16 days, the stitches are removed and a cast applied. This wait is primarily for the posteromedial wounds to heal (the plantigrade position of the ankle and foot places tension on the medial wounds where the skin has adapted to an inversion/plantar-flexed position). At 8 weeks after surgery, a pneumatic walking boot is applied, which should be removed only for active and gentle active assistive range of motion exercises with a therapist aiding the patient to begin training this out-of-phase transfer.[16] At 10 weeks, partial weight bearing can begin, and at 12 weeks full weight bearing is allowed. The transfer is protected for a full 16 weeks in the short-leg walking boot. The brace the patient used before the transfer should be worn another 12 weeks when weight bearing. The patient should be told before surgery that he or she will not be brace-free for at least 6 months after the operation.

DISCUSSION

The bridle procedure has not been used or reported on as extensively as transfer of the t bialis posterior through the interosseous membrane into a bony tunnel in the mid-foot. Through the works of Mayer,[17] Peabody,[18] and many others, the "guiding principles" of

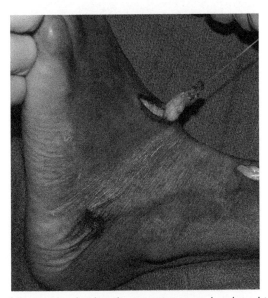

Fig. 11. The ends of the previously placed suture are grasped and used to gently bring the tibialis posterior tendon into the distal wound (incision #6).

Biotenodesis screw

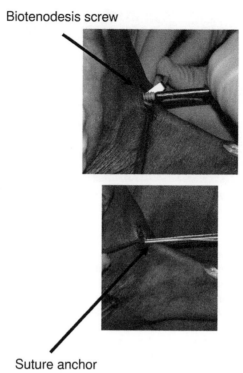

Suture anchor

Fig. 12. Both a tenodesis screw (*A*) and suture anchor (*B*) are used for secure fixation of the tibialis posterior in the bony tunnel.

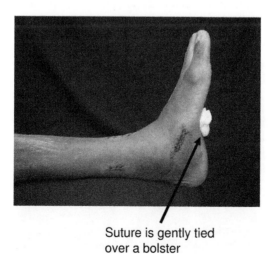

Suture is gently tied
over a bolster

Fig. 13. The suture on the plantar foot is gently secured over a well-padded bolster with little tension; this bolster serves only as a "check rein" for the tibialis posterior.

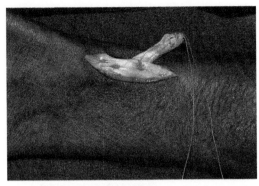

Fig. 14. The tibialis posterior is sutured through the tibialis anterior 1 cm distal to the peroneus longus and any excess tendon is removed.

tendon transfers have been clearly stated. It is useful for the surgeon to review the contributions of these early researchers when considering the efficacy of tendon transfer.

In this review of the bridle procedure, the following key points should be considered. (1) Transfer of the tibialis posterior tendon through the interosseous membrane and to the mid-foot with a bony insertion has a high degree of success.[11–13] (2) Adding a tri-tendon weave at the anterior lower leg after the bony insertion of the tibialis posterior tendon into the mid-foot may be advantageous in selected patients with cerebral palsy, Charcot-Marie-Tooth disease, peroneal nerve injury, and compartment syndrome.[2,5] (3) Patients with motor/sensory hereditary neuropathies other than Charcot-Marie-Tooth disease are at a higher risk of a poor result but carefully selected patients may be suitable candidates.[2,11–13] (4) Stabilization of the hindfoot with fusion may be necessary in patients with neuromuscular pathology (particularly Charcot-Marie-Tooth disease) and should be performed before the transfer (tibialis posterior alone or bridle technique).[2,4,6,7,13,14] (5) Although severe spasticity is not an absolute contraindication to the bridle procedure, diplegic and quadriplegic patients have not had as good results as patients without spasticity or even hemiplegic patients.[7,8,11]

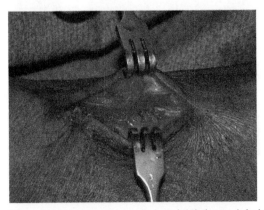

Fig. 15. The fascia of the anterior compartment is closed tightly to minimize the tri-tendinous soft-tissue prominence.

The bridle procedure as modified by Rodriguez has the advantage of minimizing tendon elongation and thereby theoretically decreasing recurrence of the equinus deformity. It is acknowledged that this complication was not commonly reported in patients undergoing the original procedure (ie, without bony insertion of the t bialis posterior tendon).[4,7]

SUMMARY

The bridle procedure is versatile, although indications vary based on the underlying pathology. This procedure will usually allow for brace-free ambulation while minimizing the risk of recurrent deformity. However, the patient and family must understand a "normal" gait is unusual.

REFERENCES

1. Gellman RE, Anderson RB, Davis WH. Bridle posterior tibial tendon transfer. In: Kitaoka HB, editor. Master techniques in orthopedic surgery. The foot and ankle. 2nd edition. Philadelphia: Lippincott Williams & Wilkins; 2002. p. 597–613.
2. McCall RC, Frederick HA, McCluskey GM, et al. The bridle procedure: a new treatment for equinus and equinovarus deformities in children. J Pediatr Orthop 1991;11:83–9.
3. Myerson MS. Paralytic disorders of the lower extremity. In: Myerson MS, editor. Foot and ankle disorders. Philadelphia: Saunders; 2000. p. 885–91.
4. Rodriguez R. The bridle procedure in the treatment of paralysis of the foot. Foot Ankle 1992;13:63–9.
5. Prahinski JR, McHale KA, Temple HT, et al. Bridle transfer for paresis of the anterior and lateral compartment. Foot Ankle Int 1996;17:615–9.
6. Lipscomb PB, Sanchez JJ. Anterior transplantation of the posterior tibial tendon for persistent palsy of the common peroneal nerve. J Bone Joint Surg Am 1961;43:60–6.
7. Rodriguez R. The bridle procedure for the treatment of dorsiflexion paralysis of the foot. Tech Foot Ankle Surg 2009;8:168–71.
8. Schneider M, Balon K. Deformity of the foot following anterior transfer of the posterior tibial tendon and of the Achilles tendon for spastic equinovarus. Clin Orthop Relat Res 1977;125:113–8.
9. Selvapandian AJ, Brand PW. Transfer of the tibialis posterior for drop foot deformity. Indian J Surg 1959;21:151.
10. Soares D. Tibialis posterior transfer for the correction of foot drop in leprosy. J Bone Joint Surg Br 1996;78:61–2.
11. Turner JW, Cooper RR. Anterior transfer of the tibialis posterior through the interosseous membrane. Clin Orthop Relat Res 1972;83:241–4.
12. Watkins MB, Jones JB, Ryder CT, Brown, et al. Transplantation of the posterior tibial tendon. J Bone Joint Surg Am 1954;16:1181–9.
13. Williams P. Restoration of muscle balance of the foot by transfer of the tibialis posterior. J Bone Joint Surg Br 1976;58:217–9.
14. Elsner A, Barg A, Stufkens SA, et al. Lambrinudi arthrodesis with posterior tibialis transfer in adult drop-foot. Foot Ankle Int 2010;31:29–37.
15. Strayer LM Jr. Recession of the gastrocnemius: an operation to relieve spastic contracture of the calf muscles. J Bone Joint Surg Am 1950;32:671–6.
16. Close J, Todd F. The phasic activity of the muscles of the lower extremity and the effect of tendon transfer. J Bone Joint Surg Am 1959; 41:189–208.
17. Mayer L. The physiological method of tendon transplantation in the treatment of paralytic drop-foot. J Bone Joint Surg 1937;19:389–94.
18. Peabody CW. Tendon transposition. J Bone Joint Surg 1938;20:193–205.

Tendon Transfers for the Adult Flexible Cavovarus Foot

Daniel B. Ryssman, MD[a], Mark S. Myerson, MD[b],*

KEYWORDS

- Cavovarus • Equinocavovarus • Equinovarus
- Hereditary motor sensory neuropathy
- Charcot-Marie-Tooth disease • Tendon transfer

Correction of the adult cavovarus foot deformity, whether rigid or flexible, can be quite challenging. While there are many causes of this deformity, the universal problem is the loss of muscle balance around the ankle and foot. If left untreated, progression of deformity is inevitable as a result of this imbalance, and generally the flexible deformity ultimately becomes rigid. It makes sense therefore, to commence treatment as early as possible in order to preserve as much mobility as possible. While this is clearly worthwhile, this goal is not always realistic, since many patients are not symptomatic and manage their activities of daily living even without orthotic or brace support. However, when surgery is indicated, the goal has to be to obtain a plantigrade *and* balanced foot, and this cannot be accomplished without tendon transfers. The foot and ankle must be in equilibrium, and tendon transfers are an integral addition for correction, whether part of a hindfoot arthrodesis or multiple osteotomies.

ETIOLOGY

The four main causes of adult cavovarus foot deformity can be grouped into neurologic, traumatic, residual clubfoot, and idiopathic etiologies.[1] Most cavovarus foot deformities can be attributed to a neurologic cause, the most common cause being hereditary motor sensory neuropathy, or Charcot-Marie-Tooth (CMT) disease.[2] Other neurologic causes include cerebral palsy, stroke, idiopathic peripheral neuropathy, poliomyelitis, or spinal cord lesions. In traumatic cases, compartment syndrome, talar neck malunion, or peroneal nerve injury can result in significant rigid equinocavovarus deformity. Residual clubfoot, either untreated or partially treated,

[a] Department of Orthopedics, Mayo Clinic, 200 First Street SW, Rochester, MN 55905, USA
[b] Institute for Foot and Ankle Reconstruction at Mercy, Mercy Medical Center, 301 St. Paul Place, Baltimore, MD 21202, USA
* Corresponding author.
E-mail address: mark4feet@aol.com

Foot Ankle Clin N Am 16 (2011) 435–450
doi:10.1016/j.fcl.2011.08.001
1083-7515/11/$ – see front matter © 2011 Elsevier Inc. All rights reserved.

can persist with significant deformity. In some situations, however, an underlying cause is not found.

The components of the cavovarus foot deformity are increased pitch and varus at the hindfoot, an elevated midfoot, and a plantarflexed and adducted forefoot. Depending on the etiology and muscle imbalance involved, different patterns of deformity can be seen, such as cavovarus, equinocavovarus, equinovarus, and so forth. In addition, a complex interplay among multiple forces is responsible for the imbalance that causes the deformity. In general, there are imbalances between the intrinsic and extrinsic muscles of the foot, between the tibialis anterior and peroneus longus muscles, and between the peroneus brevis and tibialis posterior muscles. In the cavovarus foot, the intrinsic muscles are generally weaker than the extrinsics, the tibialis anterior is weaker than the peroneus longus, and the peroneus brevis is weaker than the tibialis posterior.

For example, patients with CMT have early weakness of the intrinsic muscles of the foot. Clawing of the toes will result as the long extensors hyperextend the toes at the metatarsophalangeal (MTP) joints and the long flexors flex the phalanges. With a weak tibialis anterior muscle, recruitment of the extensor hallucis longus (EHL) and extensor digitorum longus (EDL) muscles during ankle dorsiflexion exacerbates the clawing of the toes. Further depression of the metatarsal heads results, and the plantar fascia contracts as the forefoot deforms, thereby worsening the forefoot equinus. It is curious that the peroneus longus muscle remains strong while the brevis is always weak in, for example, CMT and thereby overpowers the tibialis anterior muscle and plantarflexes the first metatarsal. This has lead to the concept of a "forefoot-driven hindfoot varus," particularly as the plantarflexed first ray becomes fixed. A strong tibialis posterior will exacerbate the hindfoot varus, since the peroneus brevis is always weak. This is progressive, and the hindfoot then has a worsening effect on the forefoot and vice versa, since the midfoot supinates and the peroneus longus further depress the first ray to keep the forefoot plantigrade. These forces are worsened, since with hindfoot varus, the axis of the Achilles tendon shifts medially relative to the subtalar joint, which makes it a secondary inverter. The Achilles will eventually become contracted, leading to equinus. The cumulative result is a circular interplay of deforming forces across the entire foot resulting in the cavovarus deformity.[3–5] It is likely that many cases of "idiopathic" cavus feet are the result of minor imbalance between the strength of the peroneus longus and the tibialis anterior muscle, leading to the mechanical changes just described.

EVALUATION

A thorough evaluation of the patient presenting with cavovarus foot deformity is required in order to understand the cause of the deformity and to decide how to correct it. Yet, we suggest that the surgeon should be able to make a thorough diagnosis of the functioning and nonfunctioning muscles just by looking at the foot (**Fig. 1**). The gait may reveal subtle footdrop and hyperextension of the toes. The standing hindfoot alignment will show hindfoot varus and an elevated arch. The callous pattern should support the findings of gait and stance. Range of motion of all joints is measured. The heel cord is tested for tightness with the knee flexed and extended. The Coleman block test can be used to evaluate the flexibility of the hindfoot, as well as the contribution of the forefoot to the hindfoot varus,[6] but we suggest that this test is used too frequently to aid in planning treatment. Theoretically, if the hindfoot varus corrects when the first metatarsal is allowed to drop into plantar flexion, this implies a flexible deformity, perhaps correctable solely with a fist metatarsal osteotomy. This is, however, rarely possible, and it is our impression that

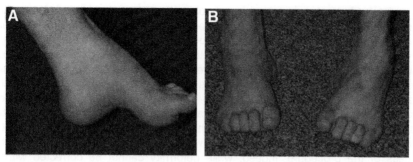

Fig. 1. (*A, B*) Careful clinical evaluation of the cavovarus foot will help to understand which muscles are functioning and which muscles are deficient, thus leading to the deformity. This is crucial in planning tendon transfers to correct the foot. In this patient the tibialis posterior muscle, peroneus longus muscle, long flexors, and long extensors are relatively strong compared to the weak peroneus brevis muscle, tibialis anterior muscle, and intrinsic muscles of the foot.

this test is overused to dictate the course of correction. Indeed it is just as easy to attempt to manipulate to heel into valgus with the ankle in equinus and achieve the same effect—that of the hindfoot on the forefoot. Ankle stability must always be checked as this may need to be corrected, although some surgeons maintain that with good hindfoot balance and appropriate tendon transfer, ankle stability is rarely a continuing problem for the patient.

Clearly, however, the most important aspect of the examination centers on the strength and function of all muscle groups in order to identify the deforming forces on the foot. By identifying the imbalance causing the deformity, one can more easily plan the correction to obtain balance. This is of course somewhat relative, since grading of muscle power is subjective at best. Nonetheless, it is essential to get a "feel" for this imbalance, and we recommend examining the patient again immediately prior to surgery to help clarify the final intraoperative procedure.[7]

Radiographic evaluation with weight-bearing radiographs of the foot and ankle is routinely used to evaluate the cavovarus foot deformity. The hallmarks of a cavus foot on the lateral view include increased calcaneal pitch (measured between a line along the undersurface of the calcaneus and the foot; normal is 30°), increased talo–first metatarsal angle, increased navicular height, increased Hibbs angle (measured by a line through the axis of the calcaneus and the first metatarsal; normal <45°), and the "appearance" of a posteriorly located fibula with a "flat-topped" talus on the lateral view.[4] A hindfoot alignment view may be useful in assessing hindfoot varus.[8] A helpful exercise when planning surgical correction of the deformity is to define which muscles are functioning and which muscles are deficient simply by studying the radiographs.

Is the deformity static or progressive? When the reconstruction is well-balanced, the foot will generally remain plantigrade even if further weakening of the muscles occurs as part of the disease process.[7] As discussed, whenever muscle imbalance is present, deformity of the foot will continually progress. Obtaining a plantigrade foot is always possible, albeit sometimes difficult. However, the key to achieving a lasting result is to reconstruct a foot that is plantigrade and balanced.

SURGICAL TREATMENT

The goals of surgery are to improve function and quality of life by reconstructing a stable, plantigrade foot with balanced muscle forces. Obviously it is preferable to try and maintain hindfoot mobility, but one should not avoid arthrodesis only for the sake of trying to preserve the little motion that remains in a cavus foot. In the 1970s and 1980s, osteotomy was used too frequently because the consequences of arthrodesis were thought to be worsening arthritis on the ankle and the remainder of the foot. While this was the case, too many feet were corrected in the decades previously relying on, for example, a triple arthrodesis but ignoring the importance of muscle balance. If one refers back to the literature, numerous arthrodesis procedures were described based upon correction at the apex of the deformity (Jahss truncated tarsometatarsal arthrodesis, the Jappas arthrodesis, the Siffert beak arthrodesis, the Cole osteotomy, etc), but tendon transfers were not considered to be integral to the success of the procedure. Indeed, while deformity cannot be corrected without arthrodesis, the correction cannot be maintained without tendon transfer. Nonetheless, if the foot remains flexible, tendon transfers, soft tissue releases, and osteotomies are preferable to arthrodesis. The combination of a lateralizing calcaneal osteotomy, a first metatarsal dorsal closing wedge osteotomy, and a plantar fascia release should be used frequently.

TENDON TRANSFERS

The basic principles of tendon transfer can be summarized as follows: whenever possible, transfer muscles that are phasic; the transferred tendon must have adequate power and excursion; the line of pull of the transferred tendon should be direct, and acute angulation of the tendon should be avoided; the tendon should be reliably fixed to the bone to allow for tendon-to-bone healing; fixed deformity must be corrected otherwise the transferred tendon cannot function effectively; and there must be adequate passive motion across the joint upon which the tendon transfer will act.[9]

In the flexible cavovarus foot deformity, the tendon transfer has 2 purposes. The first is to augment or replace the strength and function that has been lost from the disease process. The second is to remove the deforming force responsible for exacerbating the deformity. It can be assumed that the muscle will lose at least 1 grade of power when its tendon is transferred, particularly if a nonphasic transfer is used (eg, the posterior tibial tendon [PTT] to the dorsum of the foot). Although it has been stated that for a tendon transfer to function optimally, the muscle should have a grade of 4/5 strength or better. We disagree with this statement, since even a weak musculotendinous unit must be transferred if it is considered a deforming force. This is one of the reasons why so many deformities recur (ie, a muscle is not considered strong enough for a tendon transfer, an arthrodesis is performed, and progressive equinovarus deformity occurs). Think about the insertion of the PTT; it attaches to the navicular but also has numerous distal secondary attachments, which will continue to pull the midfoot into varus even following a triple arthrodesis. In the event that the posterior tibial muscle is too weak to use as an active transfer—for example, to regain dorsiflexion—then transfer it posteriorly into the peroneus brevis just to get it out of the way. This principle applies to any deformity that is being treated as a result of muscle imbalance, whether the hallux, the lesser toes, the midfoot, hindfoot, or ankle.

It is important to determine preoperatively whether the deformity is fixed or flexible. Tendon transfers cannot correct a fixed deformity around the foot or ankle. Correcting a fixed deformity must be accomplished by either osteotomy or arthrodesis before the tendon transfer is performed. An arthrodesis should *not* be seen as a salvage procedure but as complementary to tendon transfers to establish a plantigrade foot. There is another rigid deformity that is encountered when tendon transfers are performed and that is following a compartment syndrome of the leg. In these patients, there is typically muscle imbalance, but additionally, the varus or equinovarus is magnified as a result of severe scarring in the deep posterior compartment. In this situation, it is preferable to simply cut or excise the PTT to completely release the medial side of the foot.

Whenever possible, the transferred tendon should be secured with a tendon-to-bone interface. This can be done by passing the tendon through a carefully prepared bone tunnel and securing it with an interference fit using either a bone peg or screw. The use of a suture anchor can also be used. Occasionally, the combination of both types of fixation may be necessary to provide adequate strength for the repair. Strong fixation of the tendon is very important in order to allow early range-of-motion exercises, muscle retraining, and strengthening during the postoperative rehabilitation process. The ability to insert these tendons into a deep bone tunnel depends on the length of the tendon harvested, and there are times when there is insufficient length to pass, for example, the PTT into the cuneiform. In these feet, one can either pass the sutures underneath a plate if it has been used to secure the arthrodesis, for example, of the midfoot or to use a suture anchor. The difficulty with a suture anchor is the correct tensioning of the tendon, and even if the tendon length is too short to pass it into a tunnel, we nonetheless recommend using a tunnel to pull the suture through the plantar foot such that the correct tension can be applied to the tendon with the suture anchor.

When correcting the cavovarus foot with tendon transfers, it is ideal to work progressively from the hindfoot, to the midfoot, and finally the forefoot. Accordingly, we will describe several useful tendon transfer procedures starting from the hindfoot and working towards the forefoot.

HINDFOOT
Posterior Tibial Tendon

In the cavovarus foot, the tibialis posterior muscle is most often strong and acts as a primary deforming force in the cavovarus foot. Even if the muscle appears to be weak, its contribution to the deformity must be addressed. Frequently, transferring the PTT will, first, mitigate a primary deforming force in the cavovarus foot, thereby reducing the chance of recurrence, and, second, strengthen deficiencies in the foot. For example, when the tibialis anterior is weak in the cavus deformity, a transfer of the PTT to the dorsal aspect of the foot will achieve those 2 objectives.

Watkins and colleagues[10] first described the surgical technique of the PTT transfer through the interosseus membrane. The 4-incision technique as described by Hsu and Hoffer[11] is a useful procedure to effectively transfer the PTT to the dorsal midfoot through the interosseus membrane. The tendon is harvested from its insertion medially at the navicular, preserving as much length as possible. The tendon sheath is split proximally, and the PTT is passed proximally into the second incision, approximately 15 cm proximal to the ankle joint, which corresponds to the musculotendinous junction. The tendon is then passed from medial to lateral, along the posterior border of the tibia, and through a window made in the interosseous membrane. Last, the tendon is passed subcutaneously, superficial to the extensor retinaculum, to insert in the dorsal midfoot and secured through a bone tunnel. Originally, this transfer was intended to restore ankle dorsiflexion only, by inserting the PTT into the middle of the foot, or the lateral cuneiform (**Fig. 2**A, B). Goh and coworkers[12] used a cadaver model to determine that insertion into the lateral cuneiform provided optimal dorsiflexion with the least pronation and supination.

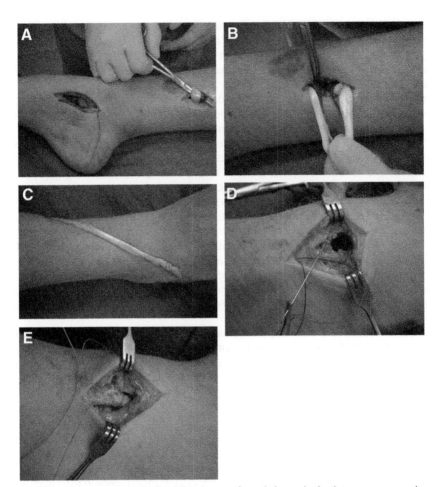

Fig. 2. (*A–E*) The posterior tibial tendon is transferred through the interosseus membrane using a four incision technique. (*A, B*) The PTT has been harvested through a small medial distal incision over its insertion, tagged with a stay suture, and pulled proximally through a second medial proximal incision. (*C*) The tendon is then passed from medial to lateral, behind the tibia, through a window in the interosseus membrane, and through a subcutaneous tunnel to the dorsal midfoot. (*D, E*) A bone tunnel is made in the lateral cuneiform, through which the PTT is passed and secured with an interference screw.

However, changing the insertion of the transferred tendon medially or laterally on the midfoot, depending on the deformity, can also help balance the foot with inversion and eversion. For example, in the equinocavovarus foot the PTT can be transferred more laterally to the cuboid to help restore power with dorsiflexion and balance with eversion.

Alternatively, the PTT can be transferred medially to the dorsal midfoot through a subcutaneous route over the anteromedial tibia.[13,14] This has been found to be safe and easy to perform. Similar to the 4-incision interosseus technique, the first 2 medial incisions are made to harvest the PTT from its insertion and then pass it proximally to the level of the musculotendinous junction. A third incision is made over the dorsal

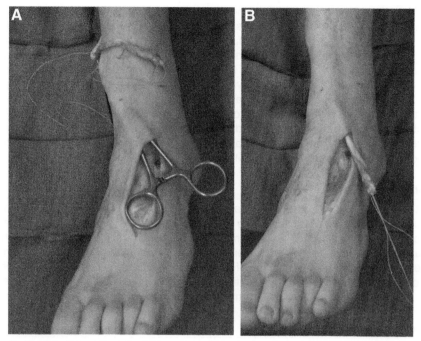

Fig. 3. (A, B) In this patient the PTT was transferred using the subcutaneous technique over the anteromedial tibia.

midfoot at the location of the desired transfer insertion, such as the lateral cuneiform. Using a large curved clamp, a subcutaneous tunnel is made retrograde from the third to second incision. The stay sutures are then grasped, and the PTT is pulled through the subcutaneous tunnel, traversing the anteromedial tibia, and delivered to the dorsal midfoot. The tendon is then passed through a bony tunnel in the lateral cuneiform, tensioned appropriately with the ankle in neutral dorsiflexion, and secured with an interference screw (**Fig. 3**).

Goh and coworkers[12] performed a biomechanical study to compare the effectiveness of the interosseous and subcutaneous PTT transfers. It was found that the interosseous transfer provided a greater degree of dorsiflexion compared to the subcutaneous transfer in cadaver models. They reasoned that the interosseous route gave an almost vertical force vector, providing optimum dorsiflexion, whereas the subcutaneous route gave a more oblique force vector, which decreased the effectiveness of dorsiflexion at the ankle. However, comparing the effectiveness of the 2 routes clinically may not be so clear. In practice, the subcutaneous transfer is relatively simpler and uses less incisions. In addition, there is also concern that the tendon may scar down more easily in the interosseous tunnel, thereby reducing power and effectiveness. Clinical studies comparing the two methods of PTT transfers are lacking.

Occasionally, in a situation where the PTT must be transferred, the tibialis anterior is strong with no deficits. Therefore, the predominant deforming force of the tibialis posterior muscle is then primarily adductovarus. In this situation, a split PTT transfer can be performed. The tendon is split at the insertion, and the lateral limb is passed behind the tibia and fibula. It is then tenodesed to the peroneus brevis tendon.

When the PTT is transferred anteriorly to the dorsal foot, its function changes from primarily being a flexor to functioning as an extensor. Changing on which side the tendon lies with respect to the ankle axis will cause the transferred tendon to function at a relative mechanical disadvantage. As such this transfer is not phasic, and the muscle can be expected to lose a grade of power. In contrast, when transferring the tendon behind the ankle to augment the peroneus brevis, the tibialis posterior remains behind the axis of the ankle and is at less of a mechanical disadvantage.

It is thought that donor morbidity of the transferred PTT is minimal. In the cavus foot, the released or transferred PTT does not usually cause subsequent planovalgus deformity. The bony anatomy and ligaments of the foot are sufficient to maintain the medial arch in these patients, and collapse is not seen[1] (**Fig. 4**).

Anterior Tibial Tendon

In the cavovarus foot, an active tibialis anterior muscle can contribute to midfoot supination. Usually the tibialis anterior muscle is weak, but in cases where significant strength is still maintained (>4/5), a transfer of the tendon may be necessary. In this situation, in addition to a PTT transfer, the anterior tibial tendon (ATT) is transferred laterally. Again, if the ATT is not transferred in this situation, the continued deforming force may lead to a less than desirable result. Depending on the deformity and where the PTT is inserted, the ATT can be transferred to the middle or lateral cuneiform.

Peroneus Longus Tendon

The peroneus longus–to–brevis tendon transfer is useful when the peroneus longus muscle is functional and mobile. Tenodesing the peroneus longus to the peroneus brevis augments the already weak eversion function and decreases the plantarflexion force on the first ray. Regardless of the condition and strength of the peroneus brevis tendon, this transfer significantly augments the weak eversion function. If the peroneus brevis tendon is torn, scarred down, or absent, the longus tendon can still be transferred to the remaining stump of the distal brevis insertion.

If a calcaneal osteotomy was performed, the same incision laterally can be used and extended. The peroneal tendons are exposed. There is often a hypertrophied peroneal tubercle, which should be removed. The peroneus longus tendon is then sutured side-by-side to the brevis tendon with the ankle and hindfoot in a neutral position. This ensures correct tensioning of the transferred longus tendon. A nonabsorbable suture is used. The peroneus longus tendon is transected just as it passes under the cuboid. (If there is no peroneus brevis tendon to tie to, then the peroneus longus tendon can be transferred directly to the base of the fifth metatarsal at the footprint of the brevis, using a suture anchor and reinforced by interrupted sutures to the reflected periosteum [**Fig. 5**].)

MIDFOOT
Extensor Digitorum Longus Tendons

If weak dorsiflexion is present and the tibialis posterior muscle is not strong enough to use for transfer, then the EDL and/or EHL tendons can be transferred to improve dorsiflexion. This will also reduce the deforming force acting on the clawed toes. Typically the EDL is used. A central dorsal incision is made over the midfoot. The EDL tendons are readily identified and sutured together with a nonabsorbable stay stitch, distal enough to provide enough length for the transfer. The tendons are cut distally. The EDL transfer can then be secured to the dorsal midfoot at the desired location depending on the deformity. This is typically in the lateral cuneiform with a bone

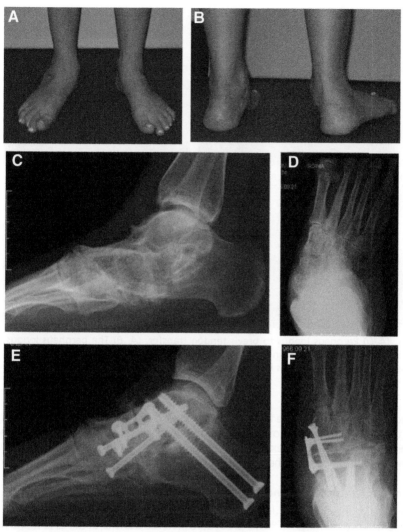

Fig. 4. Overcorrection of a cavus foot deformity. (*A–D*) This patient had a prior triple arthrodesis, resulting in a severe flatfoot and forefoot abduction. The PTT was incorrectly transferred as well. (*E, F*) In order to correct this deformity, it is not enough to do a revision triple arthrodesis. The foot must be balanced with tendon transfer. In addition to the revision triple arthrodesis, the peroneus longus tendon was transferred to the dorsum of the foot.

tunnel and interference screw. Occasionally, if a midfoot osteotomy has been done as part of the procedure and fixation includes a dorsal plate, then the EDL can be passed under the plate and sutured back onto itself for fixation. The plate will compress the tendon nicely onto the dorsal midfoot (**Fig. 6**).

FOREFOOT

In patients with a cavovarus foot deformity, such as in CMT, a clawed hallux deformity (hyperextension of the MTP joint and flexion of the interphalangeal [IP] joint) may also be

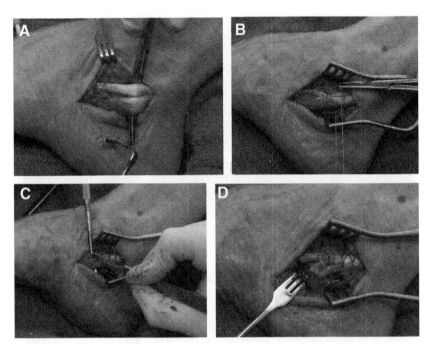

Fig. 5. (*A–D*) Peroneus longus to brevis tendon transfer. (*A, B*) The peroneus longus and brevis tendons are identified and sutured together with a nonabsorbable stitch. The ankle is in neutral. (*C, D*) The peroneus longus tendon is cut sharply as it curves under the cuboid.

associated. Again, this is due to the muscle imbalance. The weak intrinsic muscles give way to the deforming forces of the EHL muscle and flexor hallucis longus (FHL) muscle, causing hallux MTP joint extension and IP joint flexion, respectively.[15] Therefore, correction of this aspect of the deformity requires transfer of the EHL or FHL tendon.

Extensor Hallucis Longus Tendon

Traditionally, the modified Jones procedure has been used for correction of the clawed hallux deformity.[16–18] This procedure involves transfer of the EHL to the neck of the first metatarsal with fusion of the IP joint. This works particularly well when the hallux MTP joint is reasonably flexible, the hallux IP joint is fixed in flexion, and more dorsiflexion power of the foot is required (a common problem in patients with CMT). When considering transfer of the EHL to supplement ankle dorsiflexion, transferring to the metatarsal may provide more of a biomechanical advantage with a longer lever arm over which the tendon can act, as opposed to transferring the tendon to the midfoot (**Fig. 7**).

Breusch and colleagues[16] reviewed their results of 51 patients (81 feet) who underwent the modified Jones procedure to correct the clawed hallux in association with a cavus foot. All patients had other concomitant procedures during the same surgery to correct the underlying cavus foot deformity. The overall patient satisfaction rate was 86%. The clawed hallux deformity was corrected in all but one foot. The most common complications were catching of the great toe when walking barefoot, transfer lesions, transfer metatarsalgia, and asymptomatic nonunion of the IP joint (11%). Free mobility of the first MTP joint was found in only 36% of feet. The others

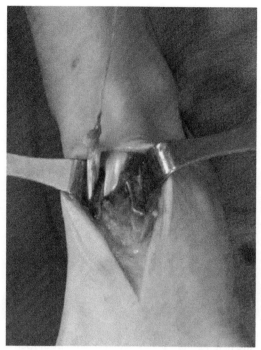

Fig. 6. As part of correction for this patient's cavovarus foot deformity, a midfoot osteotomy was used. The EDL was tenodesed, released distally, and transferred to the dorsal midfoot to help with ankle dorsiflexion. The tendon was secured under the plate and then tied back onto itself.

were stiff and/or painful. While it is difficult to separate the results of the hallux from the rest of the corrected foot, the authors thought that the limited hallux motion resulted in clinically noticeable gait disturbances. However, this was not substantiated with objective testing.[16]

Flexor Hallucis Longus Tendon

As an alternative, transfer of the FHL tendon can also effectively correct the clawed hallux. If there is significant cock-up deformity with hyperflexion of the hallux MTP joint and flexion of the IP joint, then a transfer of the FHL tendon around or through the base of the proximal phalanx can be done. This improves MTP flexion strength and moves the axis for flexion of the hallux more proximally where it is needed. Both joints should be flexible for this tendon transfer to be successful alone. First, an incision is made medially at the junction of the dorsal and plantar skin. The FHL sheath is opened and the tendon exposed. The tendon is cut as far distally as possible and sutured. A 2.5-mm drill hole is then made in the proximal phalanx from dorsal to plantar. The tendon is then passed through the bone tunnel from plantar to dorsal using a large curved needle. The tendon is sutured back onto itself or to the dorsal periosteum. To balance this transfer, it is often combined with lengthening of the EHL and a capsulotomy of the MTP joint[7] (**Fig. 8**).

Kadel and coworkers[19] provided some of the first results in the literature on the FHL transfer procedure for correction of the clawed hallux. They reported on 19 patients

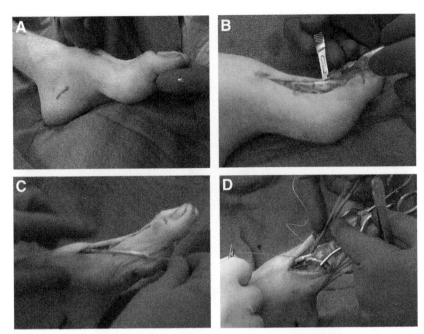

Fig. 7. (*A–D*) EHL transfer for a hallux claw toe deformity. The EHL is exposed and transferred through the neck of the first metatarsal. It is tied back onto both itself and a plate that was used for a first metatarsal osteotomy as part of the correction.

(22 feet) with an average follow-up of 51 months. All patients had concomitant procedures done at the time of the FHL tendon transfer, which complicated analyzing the results. However, the deformity at both the MTP and IP joints improved significantly on postoperative radiographs: 68% of patients were completely satisfied, and 32% of patients were somewhat satisfied. They found that the FHL transfer is an effective alternative to the modified Jones procedure.[19] In addition, Steensma and colleagues[20] published their results on FHL transfer for hallux claw toe deformity (6 patients) with an average follow-up of 24 months. All deformities were corrected and maintained. All patients in this group were satisfied with the results and pain under the first metatarsal head was reliably improved.[20]

ARTHRODESIS AND TENDON TRANSFER

Fixed deformity of the foot or ankle cannot be corrected through tendon transfers alone, and an arthrodesis may be necessary. For example, in a rigid equinovarus deformity, a triple arthrodesis may be indicated. If, however, there remains imbalance of muscle strength around the foot and ankle, then recurrence of deformity will happen. Historically, triple arthrodesis gave poor results for correction of the neurogenic cavus foot, particularly in patients with CMT disease.[21] Unfortunately, if the arthrodesis is performed in isolation, without addressing the deforming forces of tendon imbalances, then the procedure will fail and deformity will recur. The insertion of the PTT extends beyond the talonavicular joint. Unless the tendon is transferred in addition to performing the triple arthrodesis, medial foot deformity will gradually recur into adductovarus. Therefore, if a triple

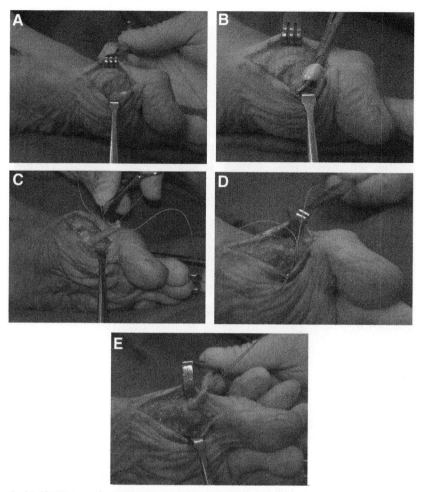

Fig. 8. (*A–E*) FHL transfer to the base of the proximal phalanx.

arthrodesis is thought to be the procedure of choice in a patient with cavovarus foot deformity, the appropriate transfer of the PTT is necessary, as well as additional tendon transfers as needed[7] (**Fig. 9**).

If a patient has previously undergone a triple arthrodesis for a cavovarus foot, and the varus deformity has recurred, then the PTT has to be active, even if very weak. In these patients, a transfer of the tendon may not be worthwhile, particularly if the transfer is to replace a weak or absent tibialis anterior muscle. If not transferred, the PTT must be at least resected to take away the deforming force.

RESULTS

To date, there are no comparative studies that show a benefit to early surgical intervention in the flexible cavovarus foot. However, it is thought that in the neurogenic cavovarus foot with progressive deformity, early surgical reconstruction and balancing may reduce the risk of degenerative arthritis from malalignment.[1,5,22]

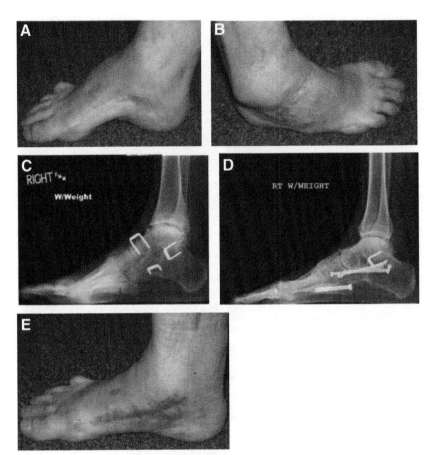

Fig. 9. *(A–C)* This patient had a triple arthrodesis to correct his cavovarus deformity. No tendon transfers were done as the PTT was felt to be too weak to use as a functional tendon transfer. This is a common error with neuromuscular deformity. However, even if very weak, there remains just enough power to gradually pull the foot and produce deformity. Hence, after the triple arthrodesis, an adductovarus deformity developed. *(D–E)* This was corrected with a revision triple arthrodesis and balanced with a PTT transfer and peroneus longus to brevis transfer.

There is very little published in the current literature on the long-term results following tendon transfers for the cavovarus foot. However, there is a study by Ward and colleagues[22] that provided long-term results of reconstruction for treatment of the flexible cavovarus foot in patients with CMT. They reviewed the results of 25 patients (41 feet) with an average follow-up of 26.1 years. The reconstruction consisted of dorsiflexion osteotomy of the first metatarsal, transfer of the peroneus longus to the peroneus brevis, plantar fascia release, transfer of the EHL to the neck of the first metatarsal, and occasionally transfer of the tibialis anterior tendon to the lateral cuneiform. While correction of the cavus deformity was well-maintained, most patients had some recurrence of hindfoot varus as seen on radiographic examination. In this series, it appears that the PTT was not transferred, which may account for some of the recurrent varus hindfoot deformity. The patients in this series had lower mean SF-36 scores compared to age-matched controls. Smokers had lower mean

SF-36 scores and higher pain, disability, and activity limitation outcomes. Moderate-to-severe arthritis was observed in 11 feet and most often seen at the medial cuneiform-first metatarsal joint. Eight feet then underwent a total of 11 subsequent procedures, but none required a triple arthrodesis.[22]

SUMMARY

Correction of the adult flexible cavovarus foot can be challenging given the complexity of the problem. However, with careful attention to the deforming forces across the foot, tendon transfers are paramount in reconstructing the foot. When the tendon transfers are carefully planned and performed, the deforming forces are removed and deficiencies are augmented, thereby providing a plantigrade and balanced foot.

REFERENCES

1. Younger ASE, Hansen ST. Adult cavovarus foot. J Am Acad Orthop Surg 2005;13: 302–5.
2. Holmes J, Hansen SJ. Foot and ankle manifestations of charcot-marie-tooth disease. Foot Ankle 1993;14:476–86.
3. Ortiz C, Wagner E, Keller A. Cavovarus foot reconstruction. Foot Ankle Clin 2009;14: 471–7.
4. Aminian A, Sangeorzan BJ. The anatomy of cavus foot deformity. Foot Ankle Clin 2008;13:191–8.
5. Krause FG, Wing KJ, Younger ASE. Neuromuscular issues in cavovarus foot. Foot Ankle Clin 2008;13:243–58.
6. Coleman S, Chestnut W. A simple test for hindfoot flexibility in the cavovarus foot. Clin Orthop 1977;122:60–2.
7. Myerson MS. Cavus foot correction and tendon transfers for management of paralytic deformity. In: Myerson MS, editor. Reconstructive foot and ankle surgery: management of complications. 2nd edition. Philadelphia (PA): Elsevier Saunders; 2010. p. 155–89.
8. Saltzman CL, El-Khoury GY. The hindfoot alignment view. Foot Ankle Int 1995;16: 572–76.
9. Jeng CL, Myerson MS. The uses of tendon transfers to correct paralytic deformity of the foot and ankle. Foot Ankle Clin 2004;9:319–37.
10. Watkins MB, Jones JB, Ryder CT Jr, et al. Transplantation of the posterior tibial tendon. J Bone Joint Surg 1954;36A:1181–9.
11. Hsu J, Hoffer M. Posterior tibial tendon transfer anteriorly through the interosseous membrane: a modification of the technique. Clin Orthop Relat Res 1978:131:202–4.
12. Goh JC, Lee PY, Lee EH, et al. Biomechanical study on tibialis posterior tendon transfers. Clin Orthop Relat Res 1995;319:297–302.
13. Lipscomb PR, Sanchez JJ. Anterior transplantation of the posterior tibial tendon for persistent palsy of the common peroneal nerve. J Bone Joint Surg 1951;43A:60–6.
14. Ober FR. Tendon transplantation in the lower extremity. N Engl J Med 1932;209: 52–9.
15. Olson SL, Ledoux WR, Ching RP, et al. Muscular imbalances resulting in a clawed hallux. Foot Ankle Int 2003;24:477–85.
16. Breusch SJ, Wenz W, Doderlein L. Function after correction of a clawed great toe by a modified Robert Jones transfer. J Bone Joint Surg 2000;82-B:250–4.
17. De Palma L, Colonna E, Travasi M. The modified Jones procedure for pes cavovarus with claw hallux. J. Foot Ankle Surg 1997;36:279–83.
18. Giannini S, Girolammi M, Ceccarelli F, et al. Modified Jones operation in the treatment of pes cavovarus. Ital J Orthop and Trumatol 1985;11:165–70.

19. Kadel NJ, Donaldson-Fletcher EA, Hansen ST, et al. Alternative to the modified Jones procedure: outcomes of the flexor hallucis longus (FHL) tendon transfer procedure for correction of clawed hallux. Foot Ankle Int 2005;26:1021–6.

20. Steensma MR, Jabara M, Anderson JG, et al. Flexor hallucis longus tendon transfer for hallux claw toe deformity and vertical instability of the metatarsophalangeal joint. Foot Ankle Int 2006;27:689–92.

21. Whetmore R, Drennan J. Long-term results of triple arthrodesis in Charcot-Marie-Tooth disease. J Bone Joint Surg 1989;71-A:417–22.

22. Ward CM, Dolan LA, Bennett L, et al. Long-term results of reconstruction for treatment of a flexible cavovarus foot in Charcot-Marie-Tooth disease. J Bone Joint Surg 2008;90:2631–42.

Tendon Transfers about the Hallux

Paul J. Juliano, MD[a],*, Michael A. Campbell, MD[a,b]

KEYWORDS

- Hallux varus • Claw hallux • Jones transfer
- Tendon transfer

HALLUX VARUS

Hallux varus can occur for a variety of reasons. It most commonly occurs as an iatrogenic deformity after bunion correction. Less commonly, it is the result of inflammatory or neurologic processes, such as rheumatoid arthritis or Charcot–Marie–Tooth disease. Trauma may also result in this deformity. Generally, hallux varus is thought of as a cosmetic deformity, but in some cases it can interfere with shoe wear or cause pain. In these cases, surgical correction is warranted.[1]

Although hallux varus may be seen after any type of bunion surgery, it occurs most commonly after a true or modified McBride procedure. In the classically described McBride procedure, excision of the fibular sesamoid creates a defect under the plantar–lateral portion of the metatarsophalangeal (MTP) joint. This, in addition to uninterrupted pull through the medial limb of the flexor hallucis brevis and plication of the medial MTP joint capsule, can result in a varus malalignment of the hallux. Other causes of iatrogenic hallux varus after bunion correction include an overly aggressive medial eminence resection or angular malunion of a proximal osteotomy with overcorrection of the intermetatarsal angle.[2–5]

Surgical correction of hallux varus deformity is indicated in cases when there is difficulty with shoe wear or pain. Pain is typically due to medial or dorsal irritation of the hallux. Several methods are available for correction of hallux varus deformities. The appropriate procedure is chosen by taking into consideration clinical findings, radiographic findings, and underlying medical conditions. Consideration should be given to first MTP fusion in cases where there is a rigid deformity, first MTP arthrosis, generalized hypermobility, or an underlying neurologic disorder. During the clinical and radiographic examination, attention must also be paid to the interphalangeal (IP) joint as well. In cases of IP arthritis or fixed deformity, fusion may be indicated. In

a Foot and Ankle Division, Bone and Joint Institute EC089, Penn State College of Medicine, Milton S. Hershey Medical Center, 30 Hope Drive, P.O. Box 850, Hershey, PA 17033-0850, USA
b Atlantic Orthopaedic Specialists, TRC Center, 230 Clearfield Avenue, Suite 124, Virginia Beach, VA 23462, USA
* Corresponding author.
E-mail address: pjuliano@hmc.psu.edu

Foot Ankle Clin N Am 16 (2011) 451–469
doi:10.1016/j.fcl.2011.06.005
1083-7515/11/$ – see front matter © 2011 Elsevier Inc. All rights reserved.

cases where the hallux varus deformity stems from over-resection of the medial first metatarsal head, correction with bone graft has been proven to be effective.[6] In cases where there is a malunion of a metatarsal osteotomy with overcorrection of the intermetatarsal angle, revision osteotomy with angular correction at the apex of the deformity is indicated. There is significant evidence to suggest that abductor tendon release, conjoined tendon repair, or lateral capsule imbrications are not successful methods of correction.[7] Recently, correction with the use of an Endobutton has been described as an alternative to fusion or tendon transfer.[8]

In cases where nonoperative care has failed and the hallux varus deformity is flexible without arthritis, treatment with tendon transfer is possible.[7,9] In cases where arthritis is present, fusion is clearly indicated and superior for pain relief. Fusion is also reserved as a salvage option in cases of failed tendon transfers. Advantages of tendon transfer include preservation of motion and restoration of the dynamic balance of forces about the first MTP joint.[9] The following techniques describe the numerous surgical options utilizing tendon transfers for the treatment of hallux varus.

Extensor Hallucis Longus Transfer

Transfer of the extensor hallucis longus (EHL) tendon was originally described by Johnson and Spiegl.[10] Their technique utilizes transfer of the entire EHL tendon. Exposure is obtained through an incision centered over the lateral aspect of the first ray beginning approximately 4 cm proximal to the first MTP joint and extending to the dorsolateral aspect of the hallux. At the level of the distal phalanx, over the insertion of the EHL, the incision turns medially across the dorsal width of the toe. This provides access to the entire width of the EHL tendon and allows for IP joint preparation and fusion. The EHL is detached distally from its insertion on the proximal phalanx. Great care is taken to avoid iatrogenic injury to the germinal matrix of the toenail. The end of the tendon is secured with a nonabsorbable locking suture and the tendon is freed from its sheath and peripheral attachments. A medial soft tissue release, including medial capsulotomy and release of the abductor hallucis (ABH) tendon, follows through the dorsal exposure.

To avoid a mallet deformity resulting from unopposed pull of the flexor hallucis longus (FHL), the IP joint of the toe is fused. The IP joint is prepared for fusion and the arthrodesis secured with a partially threaded 4-mm screw. To allow room for a bone tunnel, this screw should not be fully advanced into the proximal metaphysis. A dorsal-to-plantar bone tunnel is created on the lateral side of the proximal metaphysis of the phalanx using a 3.5-mm drill bit. The free end of the tendon is passed plantar to the intermetatarsal ligament in a proximal to distal direction. It is then passed through the bone tunnel from plantar to dorsal and sutured back onto itself after being appropriately tensioned with the toe in slight valgus (**Fig. 1**).

The corrected position of the hallux can be provisionally maintained by temporary transarticular Kirschner wire fixation or with a soft dressing, typically for 6 weeks postoperatively. Advantages of using the EHL tendon is that it is stout and has an appropriate length for secure fixation.[10] There is debate whether or not this represents a dynamic or static restraint to varus deviation of the hallux. Difficulty can arise if the EHL is contracted or scarred because of prior surgery. Limitations of this specific procedure are reduced extension of the hallux and a complete loss of IP motion.[11,12]

In Johnson and Spiegl's original description of this procedure they retrospectively reviewed their results of this technique on 14 patients (15 toes with hallux varus). Their results showed uniform improvement in deformity and pain. Average varus position started at 18° and improved to within 3° of neutral in all cases. Flexion at the first MTP

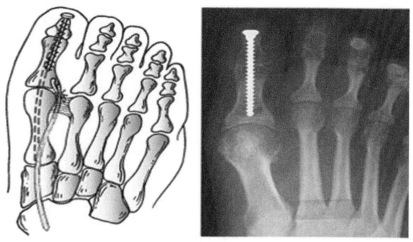

Fig. 1. Complete EHL transfer with IP joint fusion for the treatment of hallux varus.

joint increased from an average of −23° to +6°. There was no change in the average extension at 61°. Range of motion for the first MTP joint increased between 38 and 67°. Results were deemed excellent in 10 feet, good in 4, and fair in 1. In 12 of the 15 procedures, there was complete satisfaction. In the remaining 3 cases, there was satisfaction with 2 minor and 1 major complaint. The major complaint was a persistent IP joint flexion deformity. One patient required screw removal owing to irritation. One patient developed reflex sympathetic dystrophy that resolved with conservative treatment. In 1 case, the drill hole for the tenodesis was too large and the tendon was tied over a button; early loss of fixation occurred.[10]

Split EHL Transfer

After describing the transfer of the complete EHL tendon for correction of hallux varus, Johnson[12] later described a modification using a split transfer. With this technique, the lateral half of the EHL is detached from its distal insertion. Passage of the tendon from proximal to distal under the intermetatarsal ligament and fixation to the proximal phalanx is performed in a similar fashion as described for the complete EHL transfer. Alternatively, a medial to lateral tunnel is drilled across the proximal phalanx. In this case, the tendon is passed in a lateral to medial direction and tied into the medial periosteum of the proximal phalanx (**Fig. 2**). This technique is believed to be superior to complete EHL transfer because half of the EHL insertion is maintained. This makes IP joint fusion unnecessary and hypothetically does not affect the ability to extend the hallux.[12] Clinically, application of tension to the lateral limb of the split EHL tendon can alter the function of the medial half of tendon. It is questionable whether this functions as a dynamic tendon transfer or simply a static tenodesis.[11]

Modified Split EHL Tendon Transfer

Lau and Myerson[11] described a modification of Johnson's modification of the EHL transfer. Instead of detaching the EHL distally, the lateral half of the tendon is released proximally. This distally based tendon is then captured using a nonabsorbable locking suture. It is freed from its sheath and peripheral attachments and transferred from

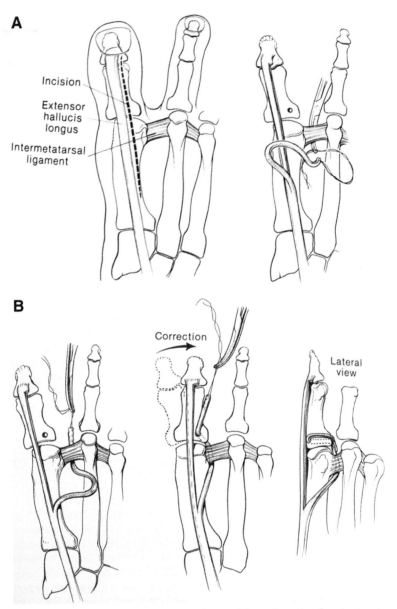

Fig. 2. (*A, B*) Split EHL transfer with distal release of lateral tendon for the treatment of hallux varus.

distal to proximal under the intermetatarsal ligament. In this transfer, the tendon's free end is anchored to the first metatarsal. To attach the EHL to the first metatarsal, a bone tunnel is created utilizing a 3.5-mm drill bit. The bone tunnel is started 1.5 cm proximal to the first MTP joint, slightly dorsal to the medial border of the metatarsal. The exit point is on the plantar-lateral side of the metatarsal, slightly distal to the starting point (**Fig. 3**). The tendon is passed in a lateral to medial direction. A metal

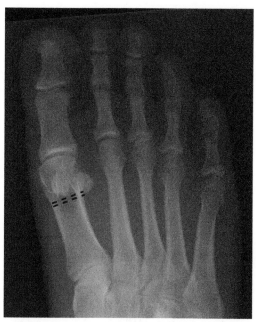

Fig. 3. X-ray demonstrating location of bone tunnel for split EHL tenodesis with proximal tendon release for the treatment of hallux varus.

suction tip is then passed through the tunnel and the suture at the end of the free end of the tendon are sucked into the tip (some irrigation can facilitate this process if necessary). The suction tip is then withdrawn and the free suture ends are pulled, delivering the EHL tendon from the plantar–lateral metatarsal out through the dorsal–medial metatarsal. The EHL is ultimately sewn into the periosteum of the metatarsal with nonabsorbable sutures. Proper tensioning results in approximately 5° of hallux valgus without significant limitation of sagittal plane MTP joint motion. The advantage of this procedure over the EHB transfer (see below) is that the split EHL tendon is often stouter. When compared with the distally released split EHL transfer, this proximally released transfer does not alter the mechanics of the remaining EHL tendon dramatically.[11]

Postoperatively, the patient is allowed immediate heel weight bearing in a hard-soled shoe. At 4 weeks postoperatively, the patient may transition into a comfortable stiff-soled shoe. A soft dressing with taping to maintain a slight valgus position is used. Once the incision has healed and sutures are removed, typically at 2 weeks, the toe is taped for an additional 6 weeks in a slight valgus position. At 2 months postoperatively, the patient begins full activity in a normal shoe. Formal physical therapy is typically unnecessary, but may be of benefit if there is significant scar adhesion or stiffness of the hallux.[11]

Results of this technique are described as being more reliable than split EHL transfer with proximal release. The tensioning of the tenodesis has no effect on the residual EHL tendon while allowing a more reliable correction of the static hallux varus deformity.[11] No published clinical studies discussing the success rate of this tenodesis were found in the literature.

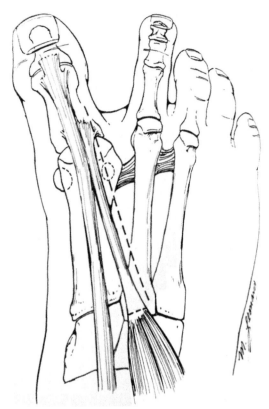

Fig. 4. Anatomy of EHB tendon and incision location for EHB tenodesis for the treatment of hallux varus.

Extensor Hallucis Brevis Tenodesis (Authors' Preferred Technique)

The use of the extensor hallucis brevis (EHB) tenodesis for correction of hallux varus is a well described technique with clinical and biomechanical data to support its efficacy.[7,9] EHB tenodesis is indicated for correction of hallux varus with flexible MTP and IP joints. An advantage of this technique over the use of EHL is the maintenance of extension of the distal phalanx of the hallux. Approximately 4 cm of EHB tendon is necessary for this technique. To harvest adequate tendon length, a 4 cm incision is made obliquely across the first webspace (**Fig. 4**). The tendon is transected at the musculotendinous junction. A locking suture is then tied through the free end of the tendon and it is mobilized up to the level of insertion onto the extensor hood in the dorsolateral proximal phalanx (**Fig. 5**).[10,13]

To attach the EHB to the first metatarsal, a bone tunnel or suture anchor fixation can be utilized. When performing the bone tunnel technique, a 3.5-mm drill bit is utilized. The bone tunnel is drilled in a medial to lateral direction and the tendon is passed from lateral to medial. The bone tunnel is started 1.5 cm proximal to the first MTP joint, slightly dorsal to the medial border of the metatarsal. The exit point for the bone tunnel is on the plantar–lateral side of the metatarsal, slightly distal to the starting point (**Fig. 6**). The tendon is then passed from distal to proximal, plantar to the intermetatarsal ligament. A metal suction tip is then passed through the tunnel and the sutures in the

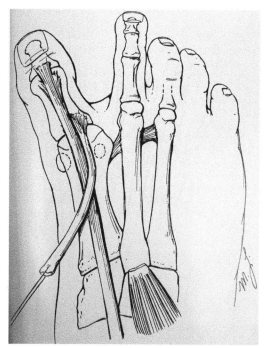

Fig. 5. Proximally released and mobilized EHB tendon with suture in free end.

free end of the tendon are sucked into the tip (some irrigation can facilitate this process if necessary). The suction tip is then withdrawn and the free suture ends are pulled, delivering the EHB tendon from the plantar–lateral metatarsal through the dorsal–medial metatarsal. The proceeding steps can be substituted for placement of a suture anchor on the dorsal–lateral metatarsal if this is desired in lieu of a bone tunnel. We prefer use of a bone tunnel with fixation of the tendon to the periosteum of the dorsal–medial metatarsal (**Fig. 7**).[7,9]

It is necessary to set appropriate tension for the EHB tenodesis. The goal for correction is 5° of valgus at the MTP joint with no limitation of sagittal plane motion. Typically maximal tension results in decreased sagittal plane motion. Iatrogenic rotational deformity of the great toe must be avoided. The dorsal insertion of the EHB on the proximal phalanx can result in supination torque on the proximal phalanx. If necessary, the dorsal insertion of the EHB is released to minimize this.[9]

Postoperatively, the patient is allowed immediate heel weight bearing in a hard-soled shoe. At 4 weeks postoperatively the patient may transition into a comfortable stiff-soled shoe. A soft dressing with taping to maintain a slight valgus position is used. Once the incision has healed and sutures are removed (typically at 2 weeks) the toe is taped for an additional 6 weeks in a slight valgus position. At 2 months postoperatively, the patient progresses to full activity in a normal shoe. Formal physical therapy is typically unnecessary, but may be of benefit if there is significant scar adhesion or stiffness of the hallux.[9]

In a published series of 6 corrections using this technique of EHB tenodesis, excellent correction was achieved and maintained at a mean follow-up of 28 months. The American Orthopaedic Foot and Ankle Society rating improved from 61 to 85 after

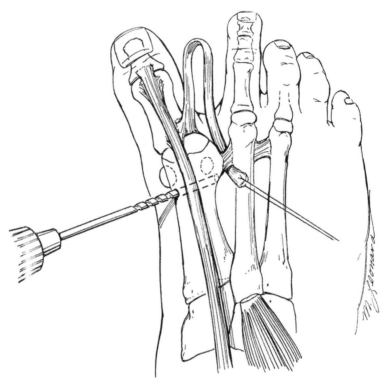

Fig. 6. Passing of EHB tendon plantar to intermetatarsal ligament and location of bone tunnel in first metatarsal.

surgery. The mean dorsiflexion of the first MTP joint was decreased an average of 10° with this technique. No additional compilations were noted.[7]

ABH Tendon Transfer

In 2008, Leemrijse and colleagues[14] described a novel technique for correction of iatrogenic hallux varus using ABH tendon transfer. In this technique, the first MTP joint is approached from the medial side. One third of the ABH tendon width is harvested, detaching it proximally, and leaving the proximal phalangeal attachment intact (**Figs. 8** and **9**). The ABH tendon is completely released from the tibial sesamoid.[14] As much as possible of the proximal length is harvested.

A second incision is made in the first web space. The lateral capsule is released. A drill hole is made through the proximal phalanx from medial to lateral, directed slightly proximally. The starting point for this hole is just distal to the insertion of the ABH. The hole needs to be large enough to allow passage of the ABH tendon (typically, a 3.5-mm drill bit is used). A second hole of the same diameter is drilled in a lateral to medial direction through the first metatarsal head. The starting point is just proximal to the articular surface at the most lateral portion of the metatarsal head, and the exit point is proximal and dorsal to the plantar vascular pedicle of the metatarsal head (**Fig. 10**). To prevent a rotational deformity, both tunnels must be drilled in the transverse plane.[14]

The tendon is passed from medial to lateral through the proximal phalanx, then from lateral to medial through the first metatarsal (**Figs. 11** and **12**). Care is taken

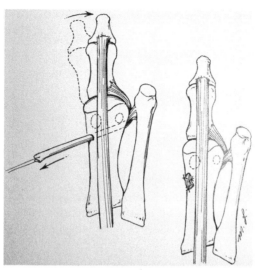

Fig. 7. Appropriate tensioning of EHB tendon and fixation to periosteum of medial first metatarsal for the treatment of hallux varus.

to avoid twisting the tendon. Tension is set with the hallux in 10° to 15° of valgus (**Fig. 13**). The tenodesis is fixed with transosseous nonabsorbable suture. The free end is sutured to the remaining ABH tendon. The medial capsule should only be closed if there is no excessive tension. If capsular closure creates tension, then only the skin should be closed. A non-weightbearing postoperative protocol on the forefoot in an orthopaedic shoe is used for 6 weeks. Mobilization of the first ray is started in the first few postoperative days. Buddy taping of the first and second toes is maintained for 2 months after surgery.[14]

Results of this technique showed good maintenance of correction. Mean range of motion was 15° of plantar flexion and 70° of dorsiflexion at the MTP joint. No patients had residual complaints of pain and all were able to return to normal shoe wear. The American Orthopaedic Foot and Ankle Society rating improved from 61 to 88.[14]

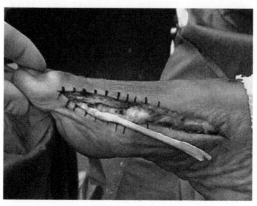

Fig. 8. Proximally released central 1/3 of abductor hallicus tendon with retained distal attachment.

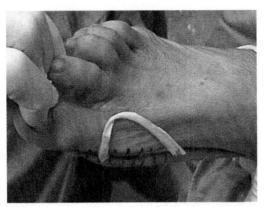

Fig. 9. Photo demonstrating the ideal position of abductor hallicus tenodesis—medial to lateral across base of proximal phalanx, then lateral to medial across distal first metatarsal.

CLAW HALLUX

Clawing of the hallux is a condition that can occur for a variety of reasons. It most frequently is associated with a neuromuscular etiology and is often associated with a cavovarus foot deformity. Charcot–Marie–Tooth disease is the most common inherited

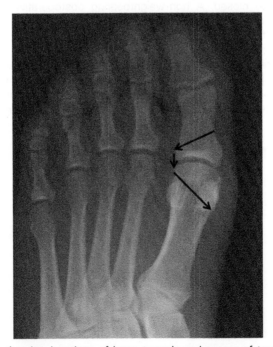

Fig. 10. Diagram showing locations of bone tunnels and course of tendon for abductor hallicus tenodesis.

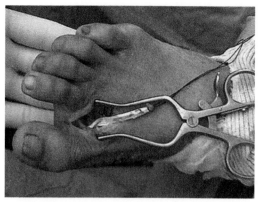

Fig. 11. Photo of abductor hallicus tendon after being passed through bone tunnel in base of proximal phalanx.

neuropathy in the United States (affecting 1 in 2,500 people) and is the most common cause of a cavovarus foot deformity. It represents a subgroup of disorders known as hereditary motor sensory neuropathies.

Charcot–Marie–Tooth disease results from abnormal myelination of peripheral nerves. Clinically, this produces selective weakness of the foot intrinsic musculature as well as the lateral and anterior compartment muscles of the leg. There is relative sparing of the posterior compartment muscles. The ultimate result is equinus, hindfoot varus, forefoot supination, pes cavus, and clawing of the toes. The early functional loss of the foot intrinsics allows the long toe extensors and flexors to create a clawing deformity of the toes. This is exacerbated with relative weakness of the long toe extensors and preservation of the long toe flexors, further worsening the claw appearance. Dynamic clawing of the toes can occur when recruitment of the long toe extensors occurs to augment weak ankle dorsiflexion. Early in the disease process, these deformities are supple, but with time, they often become fixed.[15]

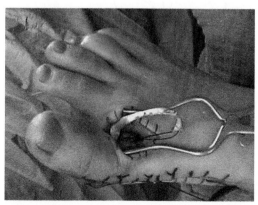

Fig. 12. Photo of abductor hallicus tendon being passed through distal 1st metatarsal bone tunnel.

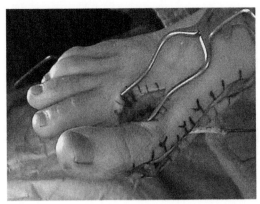

Fig. 13. Photo of completed abductor hallicus tenodesis with appropriate tensioning for the treatment of hallux varus.

In the evaluation of a clawed hallux, the flexibility of the MTP and IP joints needs to be determined and the planes of deformity of the hallux must be recognized. As with all other conditions in the foot, attention must be paid to overall alignment of the foot. Claw toe corrections are often performed in conjunction with other procedures, such as plantar fascia release, dorsiflexion first metatarsal osteotomy, calcaneal osteotomy, and peroneal tendon transfers. If both the MTP and IP joints are flexible, and there is only transverse plane deformity present, a claw hallux correction is often amenable to treatment with tendon transfer.[16–19]

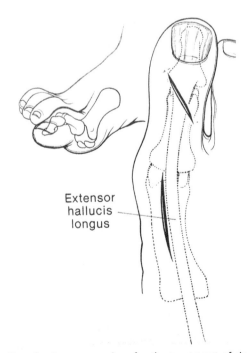

Extensor
hallucis
longus

Fig. 14. Incision locations for Jones procedure for the treatment of claw hallux.

There are numerous surgeries to correct clawing of the hallux, with the first being described by Jones.[20] His technique involved transfer of the EHL tendon to the first metatarsal. This removes the deforming dorsiflexion force, but fails to stabilize the IP joint of the great toe.[20] Several well-described modifications of the original procedure all stabilize the IP joint to prevent a mallet deformity from unopposed pull from the FHL. Commonly, the IP joint is fused.[16,19] Alternatively, Hansen[21] describes correction of claw hallux with transfer of the FHL to the proximal phalanx. This method has been clinically proven as an effective treatment option.[17]

Modified Jones Procedure (Authors' Preferred Technique)

The procedure is performed by first making a medial longitudinal incision starting at the level of the distal phalanx. The incision is curved in a transverse and lateral direction across the IP joint of the great toe, and then is curved back to follow the path of the EHL. It is continued to the level of the metatarsal neck. Some surgeons prefer to perform this procedure through 2 incisions, a transverse distal incision over the IP joint and a second longitudinal incision over the first metacarpal neck (**Fig. 14**). With either technique, care is taken to avoid damage to the germinal matrix of the great toenail. The insertion of the EHL tendon is identified and released from the dorsal aspect of the distal phalanx. The tendon is then released from its paratenon and peripheral attachments (**Fig. 15**). The free distal end is pulled into the proximal wound and a locking suture is placed in the free end of the tendon. The IP joint is now prepared for fusion. This is typically accomplished by making a flat cut with a sagittal saw across the IP joint surfaces (**Fig. 16**). Minimal bone resection preserves maximal hallucal length.

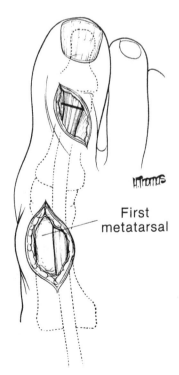

First
metatarsal

Fig. 15. Exposure of EHL tendon for Jones procedure.

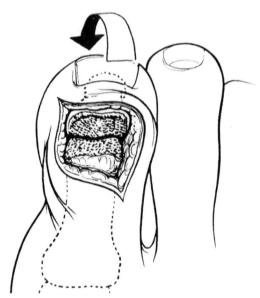

Fig. 16. Preparation of IP joint for IP fusion portion of modified Jones procedure.

To facilitate fusion, multiple small drill or wire holes can be made through the fusion surfaces into metaphyseal bone. A drill-hole for a 4-mm screw is prepared antegrade from the center of the articular surface of the distal phalanx, out the tip of the toe, just plantar to the nail bed. Care must be taken to avoid damage to the nail bed with this step. The joint is then reduced and provisionally held with a Kirschner wire. The intent of the wire is to maintain provisional reduction and prevent rotation at the fusion site. The drill is then run in a retrograde direction, through the prior hole, into the base of the proximal phalanx. An appropriate length screw is then inserted to secure the IP joint fusion. If desired, the provisional Kirschner wire can be left in position for 4 weeks postoperatively. Alternatively, 2 percutaneous crossed Kirschner wires can be used in place of a screw **(Fig. 17)**.[22,23]

Attention is turned back to the proximal incision. A drill hole is made in the metatarsal neck. Typically a 3.5- to 4.0-mm transverse drill hole is made through the metatarsal neck and the EHL is passed lateral to medial, and the distal end sewn onto itself. It should be tensioned with the ankle in approximately 10° of dorsiflexion and have a moderate amount of tension on it. The tendon transfer can be further stabilized with several periosteal sutures where it passes through the metatarsal **(Fig. 18)**. The patient is placed in a short leg splint in 5° of dorsiflexion for approximately 2 weeks with minimal weight bearing. At that time, sutures are removed and the patient is placed in a walking cast for an additional 4 weeks. At 6 weeks postoperatively normal shoe wear and activity as tolerated is allowed if there is obvious union at the IP joint. If union at the IP joint fusion is delayed, a hard sole shoe can be utilized until union occurs.[22,23]

In a retrospective review of 81 feet in 51 patients treated with the modified Jones transfer for claw hallux in conjunction with a cavovarus foot deformity, this technique was shown to be quite effective. Correction of the claw hallux deformity was achieved in 80 feet with an overall patient satisfaction of 86%. The most common complications included catching of the great toe with barefoot walking in 48 feet, and transfer lesions in 21 patients.[16]

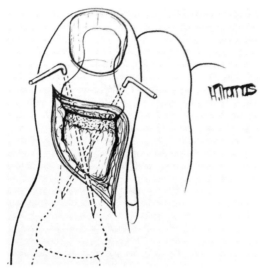

Fig. 17. Crossed wire construct for stabilization of IP fusion portion of modified Jones procedure.

Modified Jones Transfer with Tenodesis

As described by Viladot, a modification of the Jones transfer can be performed with the goal of improving extension of the hallux.[24] An incision is made on the medial side

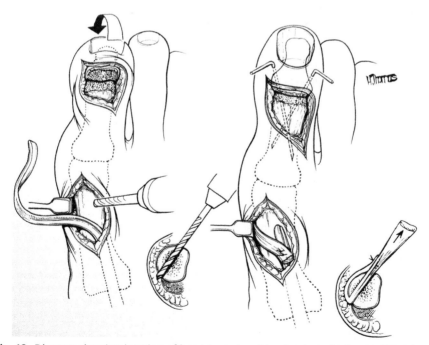

Fig. 18. Diagram showing location of bone tunnel and tendon transfer for modified Jones procedure the treatment of claw hallux.

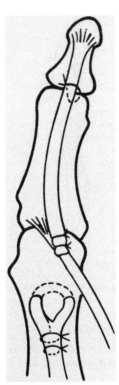

Fig. 19. Modified Jones procedure with tenodesis of EHL to distal aspect of EHB tendon the treatment of claw hallux.

of the hallux at the junction of the glabrous non-glabrous skin. The rationale for using this location for the incision is that it will minimize scar or keloid formation. Instead of detaching the EHL from the distal phalanx, both hallucal extensors are exposed at the level of the MTP joint. The EHL is tenodesed to the EHB as distally as possible. The IP joint is prepared for fusion and fixed dorsally by suturing periosteum to the EHL tendon. The EHL is then transected just proximal to the tenodesis, removed from its paratenon, and freed from peripheral attachments. It is transferred to the first metatarsal through a bone tunnel. This modification results in the EDB pulling the EHL insertion, with the proximal EHL being used for transfer to the first metatarsal (**Fig. 19**). Postoperatively, the patient wears a compression bandage for 10 days. Sutures are then removed and the patient is placed in a walking cast for 3 additional weeks. The patient is transitioned to unsupported weight bearing in a normal shoe.[24]

FHL Transfer

An alternative to performing a modified Jones transfer has been described by Hansen.[21] He prefers treating flexible claw toes with transfer of the FHL into the insertion of the flexor hallucis brevis at the base of the proximal phalanx. This can be performed in isolation or in conjunction with a transfer of the EHL to the proximal first metatarsal or EHL tenodesis to the tibialis anterior. A medial incision is made from proximal to the first MTP joint, to just distal to the IP joint of the hallux. The FHL tendon is exposed distally and released (**Fig. 20**). The proximal phalanx is then

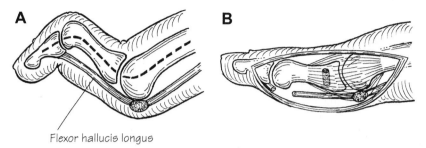

Flexor hallucis longus

Fig. 20. (*A, B*) Diagram showing location of bone tunnel for FHL transfer for the treatment of claw hallux.

exposed on its plantar, medial, and dorsal sides. At this time, if necessary, a dorsal release of the MTP joint capsule or plantar release of the IP joint capsules can be performed. In some cases, a lengthening of the EDB is necessary if it limits plantarflexion of the MTP joint. A bone tunnel is created using a 4.5-mm drill bit through the dorsolateral base of the proximal phalanx in a plantar and slightly proximal and lateral direction. The tunnel is started dorsally approximately 1.0 cm distal to the MTP joint and exits 0.5 to 1.0 cm distal to the joint, ideally in the midsagittal line of the phalanx. The FHL tendon is passed through the tunnel in a plantar to dorsal direction. With the proximal phalanx in a neutral position (10°–15° of dorsiflexion in relation to the first metatarsal or parallel to the ground) the tension is set. The FHL is fixed with absorbable sutures on the free end to the periosteum of the medial proximal phalanx and to the medial first MTP capsule (**Fig. 21**). The EHL is then stripped of peritenon at the level of the proximal phalanx. With the IP joint held in neutral position, the EHL is sutured to the stump of the FHL and local capsule. The purpose of this is to reduce dynamic hyperextension of the IP joint. This step is unnecessary if there is an IP joint that is stiff and straight. In the case of residual deformity at either joint owing to soft tissue contractures, a Kirschner wire can be used to temporarily maintain alignment of the joints. This can be removed between 3 and 5 weeks postoperatively.[21]

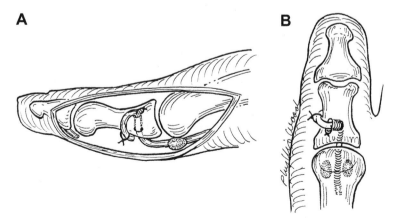

Fig. 21. (*A, B*) Diagram showing direction and fixation of FHL transfer from plantar to dorsal through proximal phalanx, with fixation to medial periosteum the treatment of claw hallux.

In some cases, a transfer of the EHL is advantageous. This can help to provide dorsiflexion strength. Hansen advocates transfer of the EHL to the base of the first metatarsal or tenodesis with the tibialis anterior. In this case, a separate incision needs to be made in the first webspace to allow transfer of the EHB to the residual distal stump of the EHL. In cases of an inadequate EHB, the EDC of the second toe should be transferred to the cut end of the EHL as dynamic extension of the great toe is critical to retain. Immobilization in a short leg cast for 6 to 8 weeks, with full weight bearing after the first postoperative week.[21] In a study by Steensma and co-workers,[17] this procedure proved successful for deformity correction at a mean follow-up of 24 months.

SUMMARY

When deformity of the hallux is present, treatment with tendon transfer or tenodesis often preserves motion. With few exceptions, the goal of the treating orthopaedic surgeon should be to maintain motion when possible. In cases of hallux varus, there are several options available to correct the deformity with transfer or tenodesis. Based on prior operative procedures, radiographic findings and surgeon preference reliable correction of deformity with maintenance of motion is possible. Tendon transfer for correction of claw hallux deformity not only helps to address the deformity at the great toe, but it also can decrease plantarflexion of the first ray and augment dorsiflexion at the ankle. Additionally, tendon transfer does not preclude the option of fusion in the future, if a salvage procedure is needed.

REFERENCES

1. Casillas MM. Hallux varus: acquired. In: Richardson EG, editor. Orthopaedic knowledge update foot and ankle 3. Rosemont (IL): American Academy of Orthopaedic Surgeons; 2003. p. 27–32.
2. Mann R, Pfeffinger L. Hallux valgus repair. Clin Orthop Relat Res 1991;272:213–8.
3. Mann R, Coughlin M. Hallux valgus – etiology, anatomy, treatment, and surgical considerations. Clin Orthop Relat Res 1981;157:31–41.
4. Skalley T, Myerson M. The operative treatment of acquired hallux varus. Clin Orthop Relat Res 1994;306:183–91.
5. Hawkins F. Acquired hallux varus: cause, prevention and correction. Clin Orthop Relat Res 1971;76:169–76.
6. Rochwerger A, Curvale G, Groulier P. Application of bone graft to the medial side of the first metatarsal head in the treatment of hallux varus. J Bone Joint Surg Am 1999;81:1730–5.
7. Myerson M, Komenda G. Results of hallux varus correction using an extensor hallucis brevis tenodesis. Foot Ankle Int 1996;17:21–7.
8. Pappas A, Anderson R. Management of acquired hallux varus with an Endobutton. Tech Foot Ankle Surg 2008;7:134–8.
9. Juliano P, Myerson M, Cunningham B. Biomechanical assessment of a new tenodesis for correction of hallux varus. Foot Ankle Int 1996;17:17–20.
10. Johnson K, Spiegl P. Extensor hallucis longus transfer for hallux varus deformity. J Bone and Joint Surg 1984;66-A:681–6.
11. Lau J, Myerson M. Technique tip: modified split extensor hallucis longus tendon transfer for correction of hallux varus. Foot Ankle Int 2002;23:1138–40.
12. Johnson KA. Dissatisfaction following hallux valgus surgery. In: Surgery of the foot and ankle. New York: Raven; 1989. p. 35–68.
13. Myerson MS. Hallux valgus. In: Foot and ankle disorders, vol. 1. Philadelphia: WB Saunders; 2000. p. 269–73.

14. Leemrijse T, Hoang B, Maldague P, et al. A new surgical procedure for iatrogenic hallux varus: reverse transfer of the abductor hallucis tendon – a report of 7 cases. Acta Orthop Belg 2008;74:227–34.
15. Kirchner JS. Charcot-Marie-Tooth disease and the cavovarus foot. In: Richardson EG, editor. Orthopaedic knowledge update foot and ankle 3. Rosemont (IL): American Academy of Orthopaedic Surgeons; 2003. p. 27–32.
16. Wenz S, Döderlein W, Breusch L. Function after correction of a clawed great toe by a modified Robert Jones transfer. J Bone Joint Surg Br 2000;82:250–5.
17. Steensma M, Jabara M, Anderson J, et al. Flexor hallucis longus tendon transfer for hallux claw toe deformity and vertical instability of the metatarsophalangeal joint. Foot Ankle Int 2006;27:689–93.
18. Elias F, Yuen T, Olson S, et al. Correction of clawed hallux deformity: comparison of the Jones procedure and FHL transfer in a cadaver model. Foot Ankle Int 2007;28:369–76.
19. Myerson MS. Hallux valgus. In: Foot and ankle disorders, vol. 1. Philadelphia: WB Saunders; 2000. p. 929–31.
20. Jones R. The soldier's foot and the treatment of common deformities of the foot, part II. Br Med J 1916;1:749–53.
21. Hansen S. Transfer of the flexor hallucis longus to the base of the first proximal phalanx. In: Hansen S, editor. Functional reconstruction of the foot and ankle. Baltimore: Williams & Wilkins; 2000. p. 422–5.
22. Myerson MS. Arthrodesis of the midfoot and forefoot joints. In: Myerson MS, editor. Foot and ankle disorders, vol. 2. Philadelphia: WB Saunders; 2000. p. 929–31.
23. Jahss MH. Disorders of the hallux and the first ray. In: Jahss MH, editor. Disorders of the foot & ankle. Philadelphia: WB Saunders; 1991. p. 1096–100.
24. Viladot A. The metatarsals. In: Jahss MH, editor. Disorders of the foot & ankle, vol. 2. 2nd edition. Philadelphia: WB Saunders; 1991. p. 1245–6.

Forefoot Tendon Transfers

Stuart H. Myers, MD[a], Lew C. Schon, MD[b],*

KEYWORDS

- Tendon transfer • Claw toe • Hammer toe • Forefoot
- Technique

FLEXOR-TO-EXTENSOR TRANSFER
Historical Perspective

The Girdlestone flexor-to-extensor transfer was first described by Taylor in 1951.[1] He described a technique whereby transferring the toe flexors to the dorsum of the proximal phalanx, one "restores useful function to the toes at the cost of their prehensile action."[1] Taylor attributed the inspiration for the procedure to the hand surgery literature, where flexor digitorum superficialis tendons had been successfully transferred to enhance intrinsic function. The effort to convert the action of the toe flexors into that of intrinsic muscles can also be seen in a case report published by Lambrinudi in 1928.[2] Lambrinudi reports performing interphalangeal joint fusions and extensor tenotomies in the toes of a 12-year-old with claw toes. The goal was to reduce the 4-bone metatarsophalangeal (MTP) complex to a 2-bone system in which the toe flexors effected flexion of the only remaining joint—the MTP joint—and were unimpeded by the extensors.

For a time, flexible MTP deformities were treated with extensor tendon releases and rigid deformities were treated with a DuVries resection arthroplasty. The Girdlestone-Taylor was a salvage procedure to correct a flexible deformity that had either failed a prior procedure or one that was found to have substantial instability. Metatarsal shortening (Weil) osteotomy soon supplanted resection arthroplasty in the treatment of both flexible and rigid deformity. Incomplete successes—recurrent deformity, floating toes, pain—with this technique led to a reassessment of the flexor transfer as a potential adjunct procedure to the Weil osteotomy.

Indications and Contraindications

Taylor originally described the flexor-to-extensor transfer as a treatment for claw toes.[1] This indication persists but has been joined by the hammer toe, the crossover toe, and MTP instability to complete the list of modern indications for this procedure.[3]

[a] Department of Medicine, Johns Hopkins School of Medicine, 601 North Caroline Street, 5th Floor, Baltimore, MD 21287, USA
[b] Foot and Ankle Service, Department of Orthopaedic Surgery, Union Memorial Hospital, 3333 North Calvert Street, Suite 400, Baltimore, MD 21218, USA
* Corresponding author. c/o Lyn Camire, Editor, Union Memorial Orthopaedics, The Johnston Professional Building, 3333 North Calvert Street, Suite 400, Baltimore, MD 21218.
E-mail address: lyn.camire@medstar.net

Foot Ankle Clin N Am 16 (2011) 471–488
doi:10.1016/j.fcl.2011.06.006
1083-7515/11/$ – see front matter © 2011 Elsevier Inc. All rights reserved.

Deformity flexibility has been used by some to determine suitability for flexor transfer. Taylor's initial series of claw toes included both flexible and rigid deformities.[1] Boyer and DeOrio[4] also reviewed a mixed series of rigid and flexible lesser toe deformities (hammer toes) in which flexor transfer with proximal interphalangeal joint (PIP) resection arthroplasty for fixed deformity provided satisfactory results. Some, however, have suggested that the flexor-to-extensor transfer is appropriate only in cases of flexible deformity.[3] Interestingly, Haddad and colleagues[5] suggested that flexor-to-extensor transfer was the treatment of choice for rigid stage 3 crossover toe deformity (deformity to the point of overlapped with the hallux) and in the setting of MTP instability. Stage 1, stage 2, and flexible stage 3 crossover toes were better served with extensor digitorum brevis (EDB) transfer. Only is the setting of a neuroma (where the intermetatarsal ligament was to be sectioned) was flexor-to-extensor transfer recommended for early stage crossover toe deformity.[5] Bhatia and associates[6] showed in a 1994 anatomic study that flexor transfer restored sagittal plane stability after sectioning of the plantar plate and collateral ligaments.

For some, patient age is a selection criterion. Newman and Fitton[7] concluded in 1979 that the procedure is appropriate for lesser toe deformities (hammertoes in their series) in children, but not for adults. Adults, they believed, were better served by proximal phalangectomy.[7] Biyani and co-workers[8] confirmed that flexor transfer was successful in the treatment of moderate to severe curly toe deformity in children. Hamer and colleagues,[9] however, postulated that simple flexor tenotomy was just as effective as flexor-to-extensor transfer in children. Their 1993 randomized trial evaluated the flexor transfer in the context of bilateral curly toe deformity. Toes on 1 foot were treated with flexor tenotomy and toes on the other foot were treated with flexor transfer. It is worth mentioning, however, that their immobilization with dressings "for the first few days" (no plaster or K-wires) may have contributed to recurrent deformity in the flexor transfer toes. Further, their unilateral transfer technique precludes the lasso effect achieved with tendon slips straddling the proximal phalanx and secured to each other.

We believe the procedure is appropriate for both flexible and rigid lesser toe deformity in both children and adults. In general, the flexor digitorum longus (FDL) transfer is used for flexible MTP deformity when release alone is not sufficient to correct the deformity. Specifically, preoperative MTP dorsiflexion deformity greater than 25° suggests that release alone will not be sufficient. MTP dorsiflexion greater than 45° suggests metatarsal overload, and this is an indication for primary Weil osteotomy with flexor transfer if deformity persists after osteotomy. Toe dislocation or subluxation greater than 30% is an indication for primary combined Weil osteotomy and flexor transfer. Rigid deformity with MTP arthritis may be addressed by rotational osteotomy or resection with flexor transfer if necessary to further stabilize the joint. Finally, deviation deformity where EDB transfer is not possible (such as after sectioning of the intermetatarsal ligament for neuroma) is an indication for flexor transfer.

Preoperative Planning

Lesser toe deformities often do not occur in isolation. They can be accompanied by deformities of the hallux as well as other lesser toe pathology. Three potential complicating factors—deformity rigidity, MTP instability, and the potential presence of an interdigital neuroma—should be assessed before surgery. MTP instability is best assessed with the drawer test.[3,10,11] Evaluation for neuroma must also be a part of the physical examination given the rate of concurrence and potential for similar symptoms.[11] A diagnostic injection of the interdigital nerve may be helpful.[3] Pain relief and

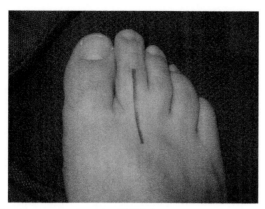

Fig. 1. Dorsal incision for approach to the MTP joint.

adjacent toe numbness after block suggests a component of neuralgia. In these situations, addressing mechanical instability may resolve the neuralgia and obviate the need for resection.

Operative Technique

The MTP joint is approached through a standard dorsal longitudinal incision 2 to 3 cm over the dorsum of the joint (**Fig. 1**). Sharply divide the subcutaneous tissue to expose the underlying joint capsule. Incise the capsule adjacent to the extensor tendons with a longitudinal capsulotomy (**Fig. 2**). Perform the capsular release and section the collateral ligament(s) that contribute to the deformity. Consider dividing collateral structures from an extraarticular position. Keeping the sharp edge of the blade oriented toward the longitudinal axis of the toe protects the digital vessels and nerves.[12] In the case of a second toe crossover deformity, the medial collateral ligament must be completely released from the metatarsal head to reduce the deformity.[5]

Plantarflex the toe at the MTP joint and complete the soft tissue release. Elevate the capsule off the plantar aspect of the base of the proximal phalanx (**Fig. 3**). In the case of persistent dislocation, a Freer elevator can be inserted between the phalangeal base and

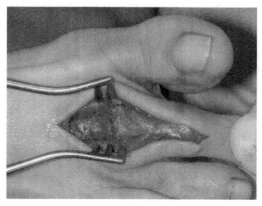

Fig. 2. MTP exposure after longitudinal capsulotomy.

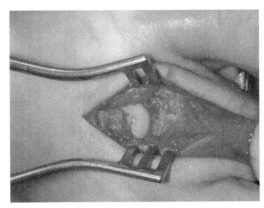

Fig. 3. Exposure after capsular release and plantar flexion of the toe. Capsular attachments on the base of the proximal phalanx should be released.

the metatarsal head with the toe in a relaxed position. The Freer can then be gradually reoriented toward the vertical while the toe is pulled and gently reduced with assistance of the Freer as a lever. This maneuver minimizes the risk of chondral damage.

The FDL is harvested and delivered to the dorsum of the toe via 2 small transverse plantar incisions (**Fig. 4**). Make a 6- to 8-mm transverse plantar incision just distal to the MTP joint. This is approximately at the level of the MTP flexor crease. Dissect the subcutaneous tissue bluntly until the flexor tendon sheath is identified. Incise the sheath longitudinally. Isolate the FDL from the FDB tendon and place the FDL under tension by threading it over a hemostat or right-angle clamp. Percutaneously release the FDL distally by making a transverse stab incision over the distal flexor crease. Plunging with the knife violates the distal interphalangeal joint, whereas wandering from the longitudinal axis of the toe with this incision jeopardizes the neurovascular bundles. Maintenance of tension on the FDL with the hemostat facilitates distal release and provides tactile feedback. Once release is complete, the FDL delivers itself out of the proximal plantar incision.

The FDL slips must then be separated and transferred. Divide the FDL along its central raphe (**Fig. 5**). The tendon harvesting process can create longitudinal tears in the tendons that can be confused for the central raphe. Be careful not to propagate

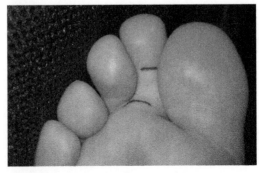

Fig. 4. Plantar incisions used for harvesting flexor tendons.

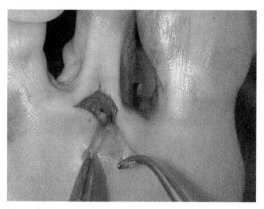

Fig. 5. FDL slips are identified and divided along their central raphe.

one of these defects because it compromises the strength and gliding ability of the tendon. Create a new path for each tendon slip by dissecting bluntly along the proximal aspect of the proximal phalanx (nearer to the phalangeal base than the PIP joint). Dissection should be carried out with a hemostat and performed from dorsal to plantar. Once the hemostat is visible in the plantar wound, the hemostat tips should be opened and used to grasp the ipsilateral FDL slip (**Fig. 6**). Retraction of the hemostat dorsally delivers each tendon slip to its new position adjacent to the proximal phalanx (**Fig. 7**).

The PIP deformity is then addressed via the dorsal incision. Incise the PIP capsule transversely and release the collateral ligaments (**Fig. 8**). Ensure that the joint is supple and that any deformity can be corrected. In the presence of a fixed deformity that persists despite aggressive soft tissue release, PIP resection arthroplasty or PIP fusion can be performed. Recently, basilar shortening osteotomy of the proximal phalanx has been proposed as an alternative in cases of flexible PIP deformity. Before removing the articular surfaces of the joint, release any PIP capsule adherent to the proximal and middle phalanges. Any residual PIP deformity should be correctable after adequate resection of the distal articular surface of the proximal phalanx (**Fig. 9**) and the proximal portion of the

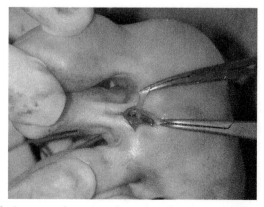

Fig. 6. Insertion of a hemostat from dorsal to volar allows easy redirection of each FDL slip.

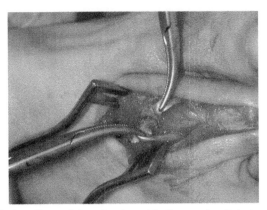

Fig. 7. Each FDL slip is redirected dorsally alongside the proximal phalanx.

middle phalanx (**Fig. 10**). For the basilar shortening procedure, osteotomy is made perpendicular to the phalangeal shaft beginning 5 mm distal to the MTP joint. A second cut is made 2 to 3 mm distal to and parallel to the first osteotomy.

Close the plantar incision before immobilizing the toe. Closure after immobilization is technically more challenging and more likely to be overlooked.

The PIP (or proximal phalanx osteotomy site) is immobilized with an axial K-wire before transplant of the FDL slips. Make a pilot hole with a 0.045-inch K-wire in the distal aspect of the proximal phalanx. This helps to guide the K-wire as it travels retrograde after distal anchoring in the remainder of the toe. Insert the K-wire into the base of the middle phalanx and drive it distally (antegrade) through the distal interphalangeal joint joint, distal phalanx, and out the tip of the toe, emerging about 2 mm plantar to the midline of the nail (**Fig. 11**). Although use of a thicker K-wire has been described, we prefer to use the 0.045-inch wire to prevent interference with a distal metatarsal screw if Weil osteotomy has been performed. Flexible pins also minimize transfer of dorsiflexion moment to metatarsal head in the case of inadvertent forceful toe dorsiflexion. Pin breakage and inadequate fixation are potential drawbacks to use of a smaller wire.[3–5,8] The PIP is then reduced and the K-wire is driven

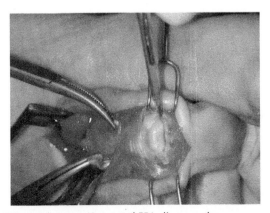

Fig. 8. Transverse PIP capsulotomy. Harvested FDL slips are also seen.

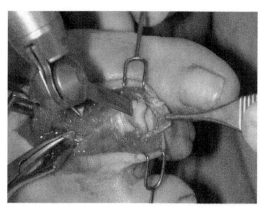

Fig. 9. Resection of the distal articular surface of the proximal phalanx to address PIP deformity.

retrograde into the proximal phalanx (**Fig. 12**). In the setting of a phalangeal osteotomy, the pin is first driven antegrade beginning at the osteotomy site through the PIP, distal interphalangeal joint, and out the tip of the toe. The pin is then driven retrograde into the proximal portion of the proximal phalanx.

Extensor tendon z-lengthening may be required to obtain satisfactory alignment of the toe.[1,3–5,13] Haddad and colleagues[5] also reports the occasional need to release lumbrical and interosseus tendons to achieve satisfactory alignment.

With the ankle in neutral,[3,5] the FDL slips are then secured along the dorsal aspect of the immobilized proximal phalanx. The target MTP immobilization angle ranges from 10° to 30° of plantar flexion.[3,4,14] Our preference is to immobilize the MTP joint in 20° of flexion. In our technique, the FDL slips are crossed over the dorsum of the proximal phalanx and sewn to one another in a side-to-side fashion (**Fig. 13**). Although we cross the FDL slips dorsal to the extensor mechanism, some surgeons prefer to thread the slips between the extensor mechanism and the proximal phalanx before securing the slips to each other.[14,15] In addition to securing the slips to one another, some advocate attachment of the tendon construct to the extensor mechanism. This

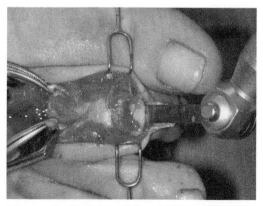

Fig. 10. Resection of the proximal portion of the middle phalanx.

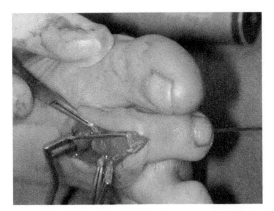

Fig. 11. Immobilization of the PIP (or proximal phalanx osteotomy site) with a double-tipped K-wire before transplant of the FDL slips. The K-wire is initially driven antegrade through the distal interphalangeal joint joint, distal phalanx, and out the tip of the toe.

can be accomplished with a few simple stitches connecting the FDL slips to the extensor hood[3,14] or by incorporating the FDL slips into a z-lengthened extensor mechanism.[4] We prefer to use nonabsorbable 4-0 Ethibond suture for the tendon repair. This knot can be associated with irritation of the overlying tissue and has led some to use an absorbable suture material.[4]

Redundant FDL tissue can be used to reinforce the collateral ligaments if necessary. Once the tendon has been secured, we assess MTP stability. If there is instability or concern regarding patient compliance, then the pin is advanced retrograde into the metatarsal head (in 20° of MTP plantarflexion). This K-wire fixation increases strain across a distal metatarsal osteotomy site if the wire does not pass through the osteotomy site before anchoring itself into cortical bone. Conversely, anchoring the K-wire proximal to the osteotomy site strengthens the osteotomy fixation.

The subcutaneous tissue is closed with interrupted absorbable subcutaneous sutures followed by skin closure with nylon mattress stitches or with a running subcuticular suture.

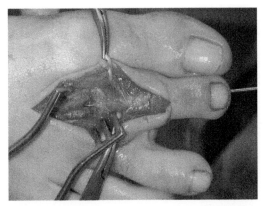

Fig. 12. The K-wire is driven retrograde into the proximal phalanx after PIP reduction.

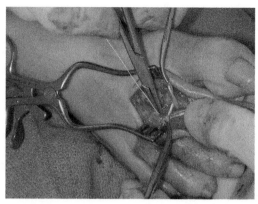

Fig. 13. FDL slips are crossed over the dorsum of the proximal phalanx and sewn to one another in a side-to-side fashion.

Complications

Stiffness, recurrent deformity, and pain are the 3 most significant potential complications of the flexor to extensor transfer. Although Pyper[13] downplayed the significance of postoperative stiffness, we now know that it may seriously compromise the success of the transfer. Appropriate tensioning of the FDL slips is also critical to maximizing range of motion.[14] Timely removal of axial K-wires helps to minimize postoperative stiffness.[4,5] Removal of K-wires too quickly, however, can lead to recurrent deformity. Appropriate postoperative immobilization consisting of axial K-wire fixation followed by a course of taping is essential to protecting the reconstruction. Stiffness and recurrent deformity are frustrating for the patient and surgeon, and can contribute to incomplete relief of pain.[1]

Additional complications such as infection, nerve damage, and vascular injury are rare, but important to keep in mind.

Postoperative Management

Appropriate timing of K-wire removal is important to minimize the risk of stiffness and infection. Most surgeons report K-wire removal between 2 and 6 weeks postoperatively. We remove the pins at 4 to 6 weeks and begin range of motion exercises. For PIP fusions, pins are left in place for 6 weeks.

Patients are instructed in toe taping and are told to continue this for 3 months after K-wire removal. The toes are taped according to the original deformity. Crossover toes are taped in lateral deviation and slight plantar flexion.[5] Claw toes and hammer toes are taped or splinted in the usual fashion.

Although some surgeons allow immediate heel weight-bearing[4] or full weight bearing in a postoperative shoe,[5] we allow patients to advance their weight bearing gradually: 2 weeks of heel/lateral foot weight bearing, foot-flat weight bearing at 6 weeks, and roll-through weight bearing at 12 weeks. We prefer the rubber-soled rocker bottom shoes, which can be used in conjunction with a toe protector.

Clinical Results

The goals of surgery are correction of passive alignment, joint stability, preservation of range of motion, and pain relief. In general, surgeons report high rates of success.[1,4,8,13] Myerson and Jung,[3] however, noted that one third of patients with MTP instability who underwent the procedure were dissatisfied as a result of stiffness, residual deformity, and pain. Taylor[1] and Biyani and associates[8] noted that outcomes tended to be better in younger patients. Taylor[1] also was the first to report that results with the little toe are often less satisfying. Finally, as one might expect, results tend to be better with less severe deformity.[8,13]

Concerns/Future of Technique

Variations have been described that have the potential to make this procedure more versatile and powerful. Hamer and colleagues[9] and Biyani and co-workers,[8] for example, routed both FDL slips around the lateral aspect of the toe in their surgery for the correction of curly toe deformity. Interestingly, the technique as performed by Girdlestone and described by Taylor describes the harvest and unilateral rerouting of both FDL slips as well as the FDB.[1]

Postoperative immobilization of the toe has also been accomplished in a variety of ways. K-wires are a relatively recent addition to the surgical technique. Girdlestone used a Lambrinudi splint and well-molded plaster (which extended from the toes to just below the knee).[1] Pyper,[13] believing the Lambrinudi splint increased the risk of ischemia and infection, relied on molded plaster alone. The technique of Biyani and colleagues,[8] described more than 30 years after the publications of Taylor and Pyper, also eschewed invasive immobilization. Immobilization was almost completely abandoned by some, as seen in the 1993 *Journal of Bone and Joint Surgery* publication of Hamer and co-workers[9] advocating use of only "wool and crepe" for splintage. Rigid immobilization of the toe with an axial K-wire as we have described has likely evolved to minimize the risk of FDL rupture and recurrence of deformity. This would be especially high in the setting of PIP resection arthroplasty.

Dayton and Smith[16] advocate immobilization with use of a "dorsal suspension stitch" for 3 to 4 weeks after flexor tenotomy. This horizontal mattress stitch through the extensor mechanism overlying the proximal phalanx and the extensor mechanism overlying the distal phalanx tethers the dorsum of the toe to prevent flexion at the interphalangeal joints. This technique might be adequate in the setting of a flexible deformity where PIP resection is not needed.

In a technique modification that emphasizes the importance of correct FDL tensioning, Cohen and co-workers[14] suggest inverting the order of FDL repair and toe immobilization. They tighten the FDL slips over the proximal phalanx until there is 10° of MTP flexion. The FDL slips are sewn to one another before the toe is immobilized with an axial K-wire.

Aiming to maximize active toe flexion, a recent cadaveric study explored the feasibility of avoiding FDL transfer by transferring the FDB instead.[17] The brevis tendons were found to be long enough to transplant to the dorsal aspect of the proximal phalanx in all cases where the tendon were present. Absence of the FDB was found in only 3 of 180 toes. Although the authors emphasize the importance of active toe flexion in gait and toe stability, the procedure has yet to be described in a clinical study.

EDB TRANSFER
Historical Perspective

EDB transfer was described in 1999 by Haddad and associates[5] as an alternative to flexor-to-extensor transfer in the treatment of crossover deformity of the second toe in an effort to avoid postoperative stiffness.

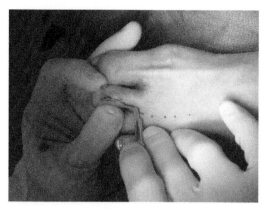

Fig. 14. Dorsolateral incision extending from the MTP joint to the PIP joint.

Indications and Contraindications

The transfer, initially described as a treatment for second toe crossover deformity, was found to be superior to flexor-to-extensor transfer in stage 1 (mild medial deviation), stage 2 (dorsomedial deviation), and flexible stage 3 (toe overlapping the hallux) second toe deformity[5] based on diminished postoperative stiffness and pain in EDB transfer versus flexor-to-extensor transfer. The authors note, however, that in the case of rigid deformity, FDL transfer provides more postoperative stability and is therefore the preferred procedure.[5]

Presence of an interdigital neuroma in the webspace lateral to the operative toe is a relative contraindication to EDB transfer.[5] Surgical sectioning of the intermetatarsal ligament precludes its use as a pulley for the reconstructed EDB tendon.

Preoperative Planning

As with flexor-to-extensor transfer, examination for concomitant deformity and evaluation for interdigital neuroma is essential.

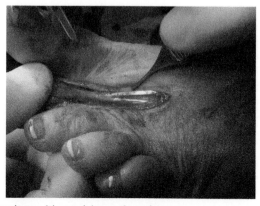

Fig. 15. Extensor tendons with overlying retinaculum.

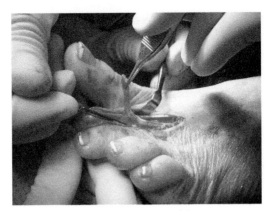

Fig. 16. EDB tendon released along the lateral aspect of the extensor expansion beginning at the level of the PIP joint.

Operative Technique

The operative technique originally described utilizes the same approach and MTP preparation as the above-described flexor transfer. Extensor tenotomy follows MTP soft tissue release. The EDL is z-lengthened, and the EDB tendon is identified and cut 4 cm proximal to the MTP joint. Tendon manipulation is facilitated by placing stay sutures just proximal and just distal to the tenotomy site before EDB tenotomy. The distal limb of the tendon (that which is attached to the middle phalanx) is then routed plantar to the 2 to 3 intermetatarsal ligament from distal to proximal. The toe is immobilized with an axial K-wire as done in the flexor-to-extensor transfer. The EDB and EDL tendons are then repaired, paying close attention to the tension created.[5]

We prefer an alternative technique that takes advantage of a tendon-to-bone repair in lieu of a tendon-to-tendon repair. We approach the toe through a dorsolateral (dorsomedial in the case of a laterally deviated toe) incision extending from the MTP joint to the PIP joint (**Fig. 14**). We perform MTP releases as described. Weil osteotomy is performed according to the same indications discussed. We release the EDB tendon at the lateral aspect of the extensor expansion at the level of the PIP joint

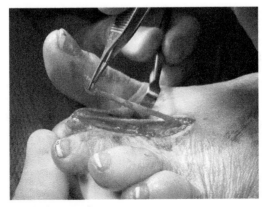

Fig. 17. EDB tendon ready for transfer.

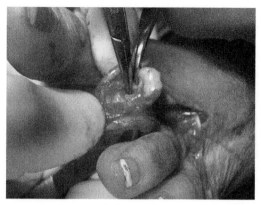

Fig. 18. Use of a hemostat to elevate soft tissue adjacent to the proximal phalanx.

(Figs. 15–17). In the case of a medially deviating toe, the tendon is left on the lateral side of the phalanx. In the case of a laterally deviating toe, the EDB tendon is brought to the medial side of the toe by threading it under the EDL. Soft tissue is elevated off the side of the proximal phalanx opposite the direction of toe deviation (eg, lateral soft tissue in case of medial crossover toe; **Fig. 18**). An aneurysm needle is passed retrograde from the space just created adjacent the proximal phalanx underneath the intermetatarsal ligament and delivered into the intermetatarsal space **(Figs. 19 and 20)**. A 2-0 Ethibond whip stitch is placed in the EDB tendon stump and the threaded through the aneurysm needle. Withdrawal of the needle delivers the EDB tendon into the space adjacent the proximal phalanx. The tendon is then secured to the dorsolateral (in the case of a medially deviating toe) or the dorsomedial (in the case of a laterally deviating toe) cortex with an Arthex Micro Bio-SutureTak anchor. The anchor site is drilled **(Fig. 21)** and the anchor is inserted **(Fig. 22)**. For correct tensioning of the tendon, the tendon is anchored under maximal tension while the toe is held in an overcorrected position. In some cases, K-wire fixation of the toes will have been performed as part of a Weil osteotomy or in the case of MTP instability **(Figs. 23 and 24)**.

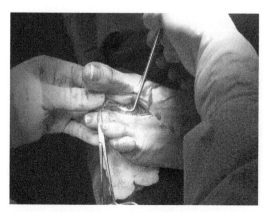

Fig. 19. Aneurysm needle passed retrograde along the new path for the EDB tendon.

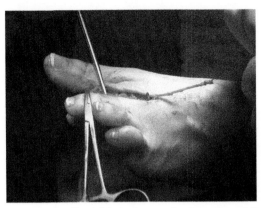

Fig. 20. Tip of the aneurysm needle visible in the proximal portion of the wound.

Anchoring of the tendon can also be accomplished by threading the EDB through a predrilled, 2.0-mm oblique hole in the proximal phalanx (**Fig. 25**). The whip stitch can then be passed back to the side of tendon insertion through a transverse hole created with a 0.045-inch K-wire. The stitch can be secured to the EDB tendon as it enters the hole in the phalanx (unpublished data). Closure is performed as in the flexor-to-extensor transfer.

We do not use axial K-wire fixation to immobilize the toe after isolated EDB transfer. K-wire fixation is sometime used, however, as part of an adjunctive procedure (**Fig. 26**).

Complications

As with the flexor-to-extensor transfer, stiffness, pain, and recurrent deformity may complicate the postoperative course of patients who undergo EDB transfer. Avoiding EDB transfer in patients with rigid deformities, evidence of interdigital neuroma, or both may minimize the chances of unsatisfactory outcomes. As with flexor-to-extensor transfer, infection, nerve damage, and vascular injury are rare but possible.

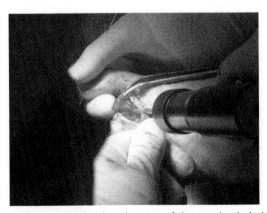

Fig. 21. Drilling the anchor site in the dorsal cortex of the proximal phalanx.

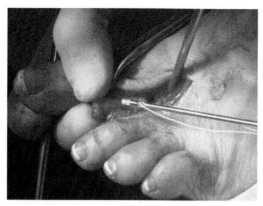

Fig. 22. A suture anchor is used to secure the transplanted EDB tendon to the proximal phalanx.

Postoperative Management

The postoperative protocol for EDB transfer is similar to that for flexor transfer. We employ taping and range of motion exercises for 6 weeks after surgery. Toes should be taped in a plantarflexed and laterally deviated position. Range of motion exercises should also occur in this position.[5] Our weight-bearing protocol is the same for EDB transfer as it is for flexor transfer: 2 weeks of heel/lateral foot weight bearing, foot-flat weight bearing at 6 weeks, and roll-through weight bearing at 12 weeks.

Clinical Results

Haddad and colleagues[5] noted a greater risk of recurrence with higher grade deformity. No relationship between severity of the preoperative deformity and postoperative American Orthopaedic Foot and Ankle Society score was observed. Marked improvement was seen in passive alignment and patient function, regardless of preoperative deformity severity.[5]

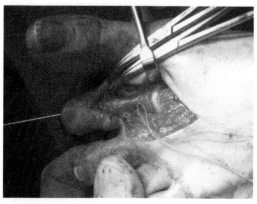

Fig. 23. Suture anchor and transferred EBD tendon in place and ready for tensioning. In this case, K-wire fixation was performed in conjunction with a Weil osteotomy.

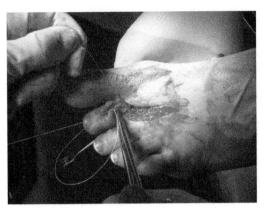

Fig. 24. For correct tensioning of the tendon, the tendon is anchored under maximal tension while the toe is held (either by a K-wire or an assistant) in an overcorrected position.

Concerns/Future of Technique

Lui and colleagues[18] proposed a modification that eliminates the supination vector created with the EDB transfer. This modified technique requires both EDL z-lengthening and EDB tenotomy. The distal EDL limb is threaded from medial to lateral through a transverse 2.5-mm bone tunnel in the proximal portion of the proximal phalanx. The distal limb is then routed plantar to the transverse metatarsal ligament and sewn to the proximal limb of the EDB in a side-to-side fashion. The distal EDB limb is then sewn to the proximal EDL limb in a similar fashion. Liu and co-workers maintain that not only does this eliminate the EDB supination vector on the toe by lowering its insertion point, but also allows a stronger side-to-side repair of both extensor tendons.

The EDB transfer represents an advance in the surgical treatment of lesser toe deformity. The reconstruction provides markedly improved control in the transverse plane and therefore has a role in the treatment of deformity where the deformity is

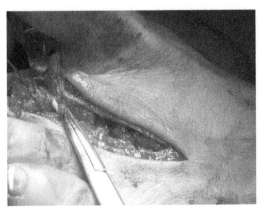

Fig. 25. Transplanted EDB after tensioning. A redundant tendon may be used to augment a capsular repair.

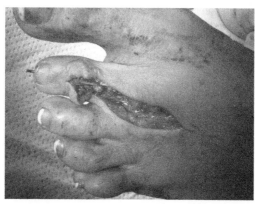

Fig. 26. Closure can be performed with in a running subcuticular, simple, or mattress fashion.

primarily in this plane. Initially used to treat crossover deformity of the second toe,[5] it has now been used for similar deformity in the other lesser toes.[19,20] Furthermore, the reduction in postoperative stiffness—one of the most problematic components of lesser toe deformity correction—makes it an attractive alternative to flexor-to-extensor transfer in many cases.

REFERENCES

1. Taylor RG. The treatment of claw toes by multiple transfers of flexor into extensor tendons. J Bone Joint Surg Br 1951;33:539–42.
2. Lambrinudi C. An operation for claw-toes. Proc R Soc Med 1927;21:239.
3. Myerson MS, Jung HG. The role of toe flexor-to-extensor transfer in correcting metatarsophalangeal joint instability of the second toe. Foot Ankle Int 2005;26:675–9.
4. Boyer ML, Deorio JK. Transfer of the flexor digitorum longus for the correction of lesser-toe deformities. Foot Ankle Int 2007;28:422–30.
5. Haddad SL, Sabbagh RC, Resch S, Myerson B, Myerson MS. Results of flexor-to-extensor and extensor brevis tendon transfer for correction of the crossover second toe deformity. Foot Ankle Int 1999;20:781–8.
6. Bhatia D, Myerson MS, Curtis MJ, et al. Anatomical restraints to dislocation of the second metatarsophalangeal joint and assessment of a repair technique. J Bone Joint Surg Am 1994;76:1371–5.
7. Newman RJ, Fitton JM. An evaluation of operative procedures in the treatment of hammer toe. Acta Orthop Scand 1979;50:709–12.
8. Biyani A, Jones DA, Murray JM. Flexor to extensor tendon transfer for curly toes. 43 children reviewed after 8 (1-25) years. Acta Orthop Scand 1992;63:451–4.
9. Hamer AJ, Stanley D, Smith TW. Surgery for curly toe deformity: a double-blind, randomised, prospective trial. J Bone Joint Surg Br 1993;75:662–3.
10. Ford LA, Collins KB, Christensen JC. Stabilization of the subluxed second metatarsophalangeal joint: flexor tendon transfer versus primary repair of the plantar plate. J Foot Ankle Surg 1998;37:217–22.
11. Kaz AJ, Coughlin MJ. Crossover second toe: demographics, etiology, and radiographic assessment. Foot Ankle Int 2007;28:1223–37.
12. Myerson MS, Shereff MJ. The pathological anatomy of claw and hammer toes. J Bone Joint Surg Am 1989;71:45–9.

13. Pyper JB. The flexor-extensor transplant operation for claw toes. J Bone Joint Surg Br 1958;40:528–33.
14. Cohen I, Myerson MS, Weil LSS. Flexor to extensor tendon transfer: A new method of tensioning and securing the tendon. Foot Ankle Int 2001;22:62–3.
15. Parrish TF. Dynamic correction of clawtoes. Orthop Clin North Am 1973;4:97–102.
16. Dayton P, Smith D. Dorsal suspension stitch: an alternative stabilization after flexor tenotomy for flexible hammer digit syndrome. J Foot Ankle Surg 2009;48:602–5.
17. Becerro d Bengoa Vallejo R, Viejo Tirado F, Prados Frutos JC, et al. Transfer of the flexor digitorum brevis tendon. J Am Podiatr Med Assoc 2008;98:27–35.
18. Lui TH, Chan KB. Technique tip: modified extensor digitorum brevis tendon transfer for crossover second toe correction. Foot Ankle Int 2007;28:521–3.
19. Sampath JS, Barrie JL. Results of flexor-to-extensor and extensor brevis tendon transfer for correction of the crossover second toe deformity. Foot Ankle Int 2000;21: 872.
20. Fuhrmann RA. [Subligamentous transfer of the extensor digitorum brevis tendon for medial malalignment of the lesser toes]. Oper Orthop Traumatol 2009;21:88–96 [in German].

Management of Paralytic Equinovalgus Deformity

Mark S. Myerson, MD*, Paulo N. Ferrao, FCS(ortho) SA, Brian E. Clowers, MD

KEYWORDS

• Equinovalgus • Tendon transfers • Peroneal tendon
• Paralytic

Equinovalgus deformity of the paralytic foot is not commonly seen, but does present occasionally. It is as a result of specific muscle imbalances, consisting of an unopposed activity of the everters (peroneal tendons) relative to the inverters (tibialis posterior and tibialis anterior tendons). Thus, this deformity is only seen when both the posterior and the anterior tibial muscles become nonfunctioning. There is very little in the literature regarding this deformity as a specific entity.

The etiology of this deformity is either neurologic or anatomic. Neurologic causes are classified into peripheral and central. Peripheral neurologic causes would be trauma to the deep peroneal nerve together with posterior tibial tendon paralysis (as seen in compartment syndrome of the lower leg). The superficial peroneal nerve, which supplies the peroneal tendons, is spared, resulting in the deforming force. Central neurologic causes can be L5 nerve root compression or polio, among others. Anatomic causes consist of direct trauma to the dorsiflexors (tibialis anterior, etc) and inverter (tibialis posterior) tendons themselves. Leo Mayer presented such a case in 1920, discussing a 5-year-old boy who was run over by a reaping machine sustaining injury to these tendons. This subsequently resulted in an equinovalgus deformity of the affected foot.[1]

CLINICAL EVALUATION

Clinically, patients typically present with a unilateral drop foot, a "steppage" gait, and the hind foot in a severe fixed valgus deformity. There are often areas of increased pressure around the foot resulting in the formation of callosities. The common site for these callosities is medially over the talar head as a result of uncovering of the talar head and the fixed abduction across the transverse tarsal joint. It is important to assess the nature of the equinus deformity by determining whether it is passively correctable or if there is an associated Achilles tendon or gastrocnemius contracture. When assessing this, the hind foot valgus must be corrected by locking the subtalar joint; otherwise, midfoot motion can be misinterpreted as ankle motion. Typically, the

Institute for Foot and Ankle Reconstruction at Mercy, Mercy Medical Center, 301 St. Paul Place, Baltimore, MD 21202, USA
* Corresponding author.
E-mail address: mark4feet@aol.com

Foot Ankle Clin N Am 16 (2011) 489–497
doi:10.1016/j.fcl.2011.06.004
1083-7515/11/$ – see front matter © 2011 Elsevier Inc. All rights reserved.

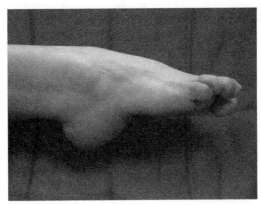

Fig. 1. This image demonstrates the sagittal plane component of the deformity, with marked equinus of the ankle joint.

movement takes place at the transverse tarsal joint when holding the subtalar joint rigidly in neutral. Also be aware that subtalar instability resulting in hindfoot eversion can conceal the ankle equinus. If the Achilles tendon seems tight, the Silfverskiold test is useful to differentiate whether the contracture is as a result of the gastrocnemius muscle alone or the gastrocnemius–soleus complex. Assessing whether the hind foot valgus is flexible or rigid is important, because management is different

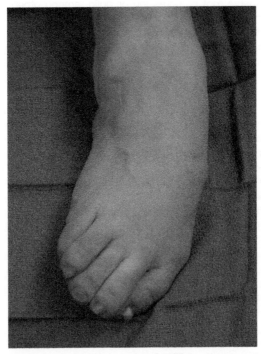

Fig. 2. Image demonstrating the forefoot valgus component of the deformity.

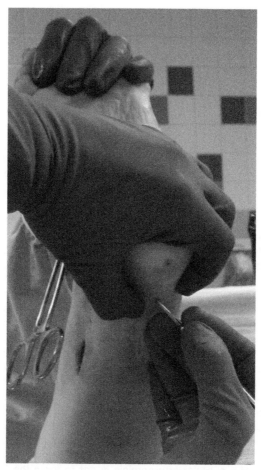

Fig. 3. The Hoke technique for percutaneous lengthening of the Achilles tendon. This procedure is used when a tight Achilles tendon is present, whereas a gastrocnemius recession can be used if only the gastrocnemius is contracted.

for each. Examine and document individual muscle power in the affected foot. This helps in deciding which tendons are causative and available in the management of the deformity. Examination of the knee and hip on the affected side is necessary, because central neurologic causes can result in muscle imbalances around these joints. This is common in patients with polio who have a dysfunctional knee extensor mechanism.

MANAGEMENT

Correcting the muscle imbalance with tendon transfers is the main principle of management for this deformity, although some additional osteotomy or arthrodesis procedures are often required. There are 2 components to the deformity, equinus of the ankle (**Fig.1**) and valgus of the foot (**Fig. 2**), each of which need to be addressed. Although the Achilles tendon is often addressed as the last component of the deformity, one may as well determine early on whether it is the Achilles tendon or

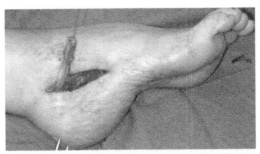

Fig. 4. Limited sinus tarsi incision for harvest of the peroneal tendons. The tendons have been release as distal as possible, and prepared with a locking non-absorbable suture.

gastrocnemius that is tight or not. With a tight Achilles tendon, the Silfverskiold test helps to determine whether this can be corrected with a gastrocnemius recession alone or if a more formal Achilles tendon lengthening is required. The Achilles tendon lengthening can be done either percutaneously as described by Hoke[2] (**Fig. 3**) or as an open z-lengthening.[3]

Although the hind foot valgus is not corrected at this stage, one should consider not only the muscle imbalance, but also any fixed hind foot valgus deformity itself, because this affects the incisions to be used. If the hind foot valgus is passively correctable, a decision needs to be made whether the subtalar joint is stable or unstable. Mayer[1] highlighted this in his article discussing the approach to the paralytic foot. In cases where the subtalar joint is stable, a medial sliding calcaneal osteotomy is advisable to help correct the valgus deformity.[4] However, if the subtalar joint is unstable, a subtalar fusion is required. This was first described by Hoke in 1921.[2] Leo Mayer[1] mentions this as being the solution to securing a permanent correction in the paralytic foot. In children, it is better to perform a Grice procedure (extra-articular fusion), which was first described in 1945.[5,6] Instead of a subtalar fusion in the young patient, an arthroereisis screw can be considered, although this must be used correctly. The goal of a subtalar arthroereisis is not to force the foot into a neutral position, but because of the pressure of the implant in the sinus tarsi, it functions through proprioception to prevent the heel from going into valgus and finally through

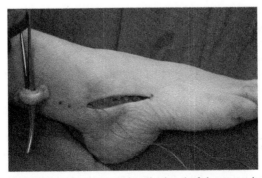

Fig. 5. Proximal lateral incision demonstrated at the level of the musculotendinous junction, with the peroneal tendons being delivered from the sinus tarsi incision into the proximal incision.

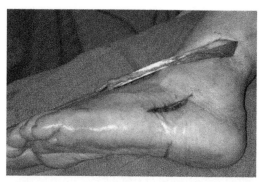

Fig. 6. Demonstration of the proposed vector of the peroneal tendon transfer, as well as confirmation of adequate length of the transferred tendons.

adaption to realign the hind foot more permanently.[7] When the hindfoot deformity is rigid, a subtalar arthrodesis with deformity correction is required. The hindfoot valgus is only 1 component of the deformity, and not infrequently, there is abduction across the transverse tarsal joint as a result of the constant pull of the peroneus brevis, and a triple arthrodesis is required.

Regardless of the bony procedures planned, a tendon transfer is always required to correct the hindfoot valgus as well as restore ankle dorsiflexion. Not infrequently, the only functioning muscles are the peroneals, and generally we transfer both of these tendons. Mayer and Biesalski were pioneers in tendon transfer surgery, and first published their work on the physiology of tendon transplantation in 1916.[8] In this article, they published the cardinal principles of tendon transplantation, some of which are still adhered to today. In a follow-up article in 1936, Mayer discusses the management of the paralytic equinovalgus foot. He describes the transfer of peroneus longus through the anterior tibial tendon sheath (so-called physiologic method) and inserting it through a split in the anterior tibial tendon into the medial cuneiform. The reason he proposed keeping the peroneus longus in the anterior tibial tendon sheath was to benefit from the gliding mechanism of the paralyzed tendon, which he called physiologic. The peroneus brevis was then transferred subcutaneously to the base of the fourth metatarsal, through a drill hole.[1] We do not use this treatment method, and as described below, find it far easier to transfer the tendons "over the

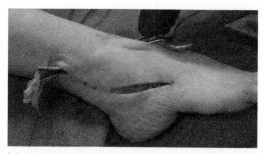

Fig. 7. Clamp placed through subcutaneous tunnel to deliver the peroneal tendons from the lateral compartment to the dorsum of the midfoot. This path is superficial to the extensor retinaculum.

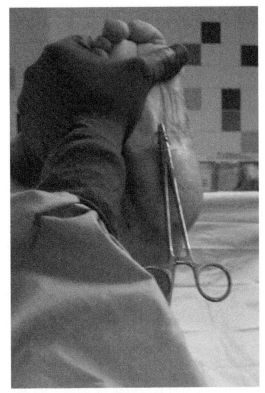

Fig. 8. With the foot being held in dorsiflexion, the transferred tendons are tensioned by advancing the sutures through the plantar surface of the foot, and held at that tension with a needle driver to allow for final fixation with a biotenodesis screw and/or suture anchor.

top" of the fibula. Occasionally, the extensor hallucis longus or the extensor digitorum longus are functioning, and these too can be used to balance the foot and improve dorsiflexion. However, the mainstay of the procedure is to rebalance and power the hindfoot by virtue of the transfer of the peroneals.

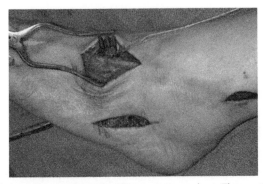

Fig. 9. The transfer can be reinforced with a suture anchor. The resting tension of the transfer can be seen along it's subcutaneous path.

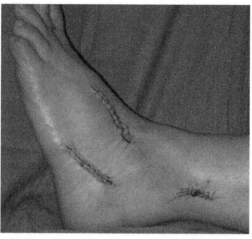

Fig. 10. Final resting position of the foot following tendon transfer and Achilles lengthening.

Our treatment for paralytic equinovalgus deformity consists of transferring both peroneal tendons over the anterior fibula to the lateral cuneiform. Theoretically, one could consider transfer of the brevis tendon only to offset the valgus deformity and provide a functioning muscle to dorsiflex the foot. The advantage of leaving the functioning peroneus longus behind is to maintain the position of the first metatarsal, but if the first tarsometatarsal joint is unstable an arthrodesis of the joint is preferable and the peroneus longus used to augment dorsiflexion strength.

Depending on the need for a calcaneus osteotomy or a subtalar arthrodesis, the length of the lateral incision can be quite short over the lateral border of the foot, just plantar to the sinus tarsi to cut the tendons as far distally as possible (**Fig. 4**). A second incision is made more proximally, just posterior to the fibula near the level of the musculotendinous junction. The tendons are delivered subcutaneously into the proximal wound, and are then secured with a nonresorbable suture (**Fig. 5**). The reason for this more proximal incision is so that the pull of the transferred tendons will be in a straighter line, thus maximizing the function (**Fig. 6**). It is very important to completely free up the lateral fascia and retinaculum such that there is no block to the passage of the peroneals over the anterior fibula to the foot. There must be no

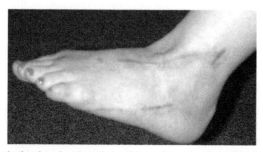

Fig. 11. Post-operatively, the plantigrade position of the foot is maintained by the function of the transferred tendons.

angulation of the tendons, which should pass smoothly over the fibula. A third incision is then made over the dorsum of the midfoot. Most of the time the tendons are inserted into the lateral cuneiform, but the ultimate point of insertion depends on the deformity and residual surrounding muscle function. The lateral cuneiform represents the midpoint of the midfoot, but if for example there remains slight function of either the anterior or posterior tibial muscle, then the peroneal tendons can be transferred more laterally into the cuboid. Careful dissection is made through the soft tissue protecting the branches of the superficial peroneal nerve. The extensor tendons are then retracted and the periosteum overlying the lateral cuneiform is incised, and the tendons are then routed anterior to the fibula and passed subcutaneously to their insertion point in the lateral cuneiform. This is done by using a long, curved clamp that must pass subcutaneously from the dorsal incision over the anterolateral aspect of the leg (**Fig. 7**). If the tendons are passed under the retinaculum, they eventually get stuck. The suture ends are then grasped and the tendons delivered into the dorsal incision.

Fixation of the transfer can be performed with multiple techniques. Our preference is to use a combination of suture anchor and a bone plug or interference screw for fixation. A guide wire is placed through the center of the lateral cuneiform. The position of the guide wire is confirmed using multiplanar fluoroscopic images. The tendons' combined diameter is measured, the guide wire is removed, and an appropriate diameter gouge or trephine used to remove a bone plug, which is of slightly smaller diameter than the tendons. A suture anchor is then inserted into the cancellous bone in the side of the tunnel. The sutures in the tendons are threaded through the eye of a Beath needle, the needle then advanced through the cuneiform and out the plantar surface of the foot. With the ankle in 10° of dorsiflexion the tendons are tensioned appropriately, at almost maximal elongation (**Fig. 8**). The fiber wire anchor sutures are then used to secure the tendon in the tunnel by placing the suture into both sides of the tendon with 1 limb of the suture and tying it to the other limb at the anchor insertion site. The previously harvested bone plug is then reinserted into the tunnel against the tendons as further fixation (**Fig. 9**). After adequate fixation, the tendon and sutures are simply cut flush with the skin on the plantar surface of the foot (**Fig. 10**).[4,9]

If additional dorsiflexion power is required the extensor hallucis longus, the extensor digitorum longus, or both, if functioning can be transferred to the first metatarsal or anywhere in the midfoot. If the first metatarsal is unstable at the tarsometatarsal joint, and the surgery is performed in a younger patient, it may be necessary to perform an arthrodesis of the first tarsometatarsal joint to prevent the development of metatarsus elevatus with a dorsal bunion. The extensor digitorum longus tendons are also available for transfer proximally.

Depending on the procedure or combination of procedures that are performed, a period of immobilization and protected weight bearing is indicated, for up to 6 weeks. Generally, if all that is performed is the tendon transfer with stable fixation, bearing of weight in a boot is permitted at 2 weeks. Permanent deformity correction and some active dorsiflexion is the desired end result (**Fig. 11**).

SUMMARY

The correction of the paralytic equinovalgus deformity is a challenging problem that, when preformed well, can be satisfying for both surgeon and patient. The goals of treatment are to create a stable, plantigrade, and functional foot that does not require bracing. It is important to adhere to the basic principles of tendon transfer. Make the patient aware that intensive muscle retraining is required in the rehabilitation phase.

With careful preoperative planning, appropriate bony procedures, and functional tendon transfers, good results are achievable.

REFERENCES

1. Mayer L. The physiological method of tendon transplantation in the treatment of paralytic drop foot. J Bone Joint Surg 1937;19:389.
2. Hoke, M. An operation for stabilizing paralytic feet. J Bone Joint Surg Am 1921;3:494–507.
3. Hatt RN, Lamphier TA. Triple hemisection: a simplified procedure for lengthening the Achilles tendon. N Engl J Med 1947;236:166–9.
4. Myerson MS. Tendon transfers for management of paralytic deformity. In: Reconstructive foot and ankle surgery: management of complications. 2nd edition. Philadelphia: Saunders; 2010. p. 175–90.
5. Watts HG. Orthopedic techniques in the management of the residua of paralytic poliomyelitis. Techniques in Orthopaedics 2005;20:179–89.
6. Grice DS. An extra-articular arthrodesis of the subastragalar joint for correction of paralytic flat feet in children. J Bone Joint Surg 1952;34A:927–40.
7. Crawford AH, Kucharzyk D, Roy DR, et al. Subtalar stabilization of the planovalgus foot by staple arthroereisis in young children who have neuromuscular problems. J Bone Joint Surg Am 1990;72:840–5.
8. Biesalski K, Mayer L. Die physiologische Sehnenverpflanzung. Berlin: Julius Springer; 1916.
9. Jeng C, Myerson MS. The uses of tendon transfers to correct paralytic deformity of the foot and ankle. Foot Ankle Clin North Am 2004;320:319–37.

The Management of Spastic Equinovarus Deformity Following Stroke and Head Injury

Mary Ann Keenan, MD

KEYWORDS

- Equinovarus deformity
- Split anterior tibialis tendon transfer (SPLATT) • Foot deformity

Spastic equinovarus (SEV) foot deformity is common in patients with upper motor neuron syndrome (UMNS) following stroke and traumatic brain injury. UMNS is characterized by muscle weakness, spasticity (an exaggerated response to a quick stretch stimulus), associated movements (synkinesis), and abnormal patterns of muscle activation.[1] The equinovarus posture of the foot causes significant problems with shoe wear, standing, transfers, and walking (**Fig. 1**).[2–8] The deformity often cannot be managed with nonsurgical treatments such as chemodenervation, orthoses, and physical therapy. In fact, these nonsurgical treatment modalities, when attempted for long periods of time, are more costly and less effective than surgical treatment.[9]

Equinovarus deformity is the result of abnormal activity in multiple muscles.[10–13] To address SEV deformity, a constellation of procedures may be used, including the split anterior tibial tendon transfer (SPLATT), Achilles lengthening, flexor digitorum longus (FDL) transfer to the calcaneus, and/or extensor hallucis longus transfer to the middle cuneiform.[14–22] The goal of these procedures is to establish a more functional, plantigrade foot. The choice of tendon transfers must be tailored to the individual patient, depending on the nature, severity, and suppleness of deformity, as well as functional status and patient expectations.

The correction of an SEV foot requires careful preoperative planning to determine which muscles are contributing to the deformity. Laboratory gait analysis with dynamic polyelectromyography is very useful and the gold standard for assessment (**Fig. 2**).[10–12,23] Gait analysis, however, is not always available. A clinical evaluation, done with care and knowledge of the common muscle imbalances, can provide the

No external funding was received for preparation of this manuscript. The author has no financial conflicts of interest to report. The author retains copyright for all illustrations.

Department of Orthopaedic Surgery, University of Pennsylvania School of Medicine, 3400 Spruce Street, 2 Silverstien Pavillion, Philadelphia, PA 19104, USA

E-mail address: MaryAnn.Keenan@uphs.upenn.edu

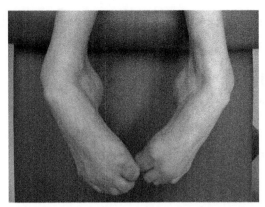

Fig. 1. Patient with an SEV foot secondary to traumatic brain injury. There is marked inversion of the heel secondary to overactivity of the tibialis posterior muscle.

surgeon with sufficient information to make an appropriate decision regarding the tendon transfers and lengthenings needed to correct the foot deformity.

This article presents the evaluation and surgical techniques of combined multitendon transfers and lengthenings for correction of SEV deformity. These tendon transfers reliably result in correction of the equinovarus deformity with a plantigrade foot, functional improvements in ambulation and progression with ambulatory aids, and improvement in quality of life.

TIMING OF SURGERY

Recovery of motor function after an upper motor neuron insult such as stroke or traumatic brain injury can continue for up to 6 to 9 months. For this reason it is recommended to defer surgery for correction of deformity, spasticity, or contractures until after this period. No prospective study has determined specific criteria for surgical versus nonsurgical treatment of SEV deformity, including potential timing and thresholds for surgical intervention. Namdari and colleagues investigated outcomes of the SPLATT procedure in a cohort of patients with poststroke SEV deformity and reported that sex and age did not significantly influence outcomes.[24] Patients experienced significant benefits from surgery regardless of time from stroke to surgery (range, 16–500 months). Conclusions could not be drawn from this data to determine if earlier surgery would have resulted in improved outcomes.

PREOPERATIVE EVALUATION

Preoperative evaluation is useful to categorize patients into ambulatory and nonambulatory groups. Both ambulatory and nonambulatory patients can benefit from surgery to provide a plantigrade foot that allows better sitting balance and more comfortable fit into a brace or shoe. It is also possible that improved brace wear and comfort may allow a nonambulatory patient to ambulate.

When considering surgery, the components of the SEV deformity must be evaluated carefully. Thorough clinical evaluation, laboratory gait analysis, and dynamic polyelectromyography are most helpful.[10–12,23]

Clinically, the degree of dynamic deformity must be assessed and delineated from fixed soft tissue and joint contractures, or bony deformity. Spasticity is dynamic,

Gait & Motion Analysis Laboratory

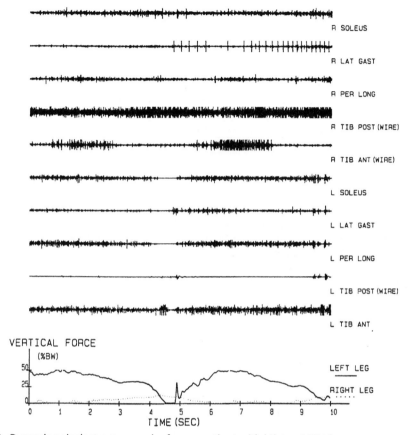

Fig. 2. Dynamic polyelectromyography from a patient with bilateral SEV feet.

related to body position and movement, and affected by various stimuli. A cold examining room, loud noises, difficult movements, and other stresses exacerbate muscle tone and elicit stereotypical patterns of movement. As much as possible, a patient should be examined in multiple positions and observed during various activities. Observing the position of the foot during transfers and while removing shoes and socks provides excellent opportunities for clinical assessment. Even a nonambulatory patient should be observed in an upright position whenever possible. Associated reactions (synkinesis) are common in UMNS. (Synkinesis refers to involuntary activity in one limb that is associated with a voluntary movement effort made in other limbs.[25])

Physical examination should include both active and passive movements performed in a sitting position. The degree of muscle tone can be rated using the Modified Ashworth Scale (**Table 1**). The Modified Ashworth Scale is a practical clinical instrument for measuring spasticity and has been shown to be both reliable and repeatable.[26–28]

Asking a patient to flex and extend the knee while sitting on an examination table may show hyperextension of the great toe (**Fig. 3**). This indicates that the extensor hallucis

Table 1
Modified Ashworth Scale for grading spasticity

Grade	Description
0	No increase in muscle tone throughout flexion or extension movement
1	Slight increase in muscle tone manifested by a catch and release at the end of the range of motion when the limb is moved into flexion or extension
1+	Slight increase in muscle tone, manifested by a catch, followed by minimal resistance throughout the remainder (<50%) of range of motion
2	More marked increase in muscle tone through most of the range of motion, but the affected limb is easily moved
3	Considerable increase in muscle tone; passive movement is difficult
4	Affected limb is rigid in flexion and extension

From Refs.[26–28]

longus (EHL) is contributing to the varus. During standing and walking, the activity of the EHL may be masked by the stronger pull of the flexor hallucis longus (FHL). Most often the activity of the tibialis anterior muscle is obvious, with the tendon appearing prominent in conjunction with a varus posture of the forefoot. When there is significant inversion of the heel, the tibialis posterior is likely contributing to the deformity.

Equinus deformity generally is the result of abnormal activity of the gastrocnemius, soleus, FDL, and FHL muscles. Comparison of ankle dorsiflexion with the knee

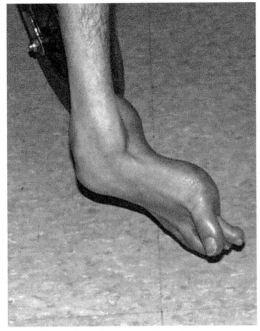

Fig. 3. A Patient with an SEV foot and hyperextension of the hallux secondary to overactivity of the extensor hallucis longus (EHL) muscle.

Table 2 Functional Ambulation Scale	
Level	**Status of Ambulation**
0	Nonambulatory
1	Nonfunctional ambulation
2	Household ambulation
3	Neighborhood ambulation
4	Independent community ambulation
5	Normal ambulation

Data from Viosca E, Martinez JL, Almagro PL, et al. Proposal and validation of a new functional ambulation classification scale for clinical use. Arch Phys Med Rehabil 2005;86:1234–8.

extended and flexed is not a reliable method of distinguishing the relative dynamic (spastic) contributions of the gastrocnemius and soleus muscles, because knee extension triggers a mass pattern of activity in the entire leg, including the ankle plantarflexors and long toe flexor muscles.[29,30] When dealing with a static (nonspastic) equinus deformity, flexion of the knee resulting in improved ankle dorsiflexion can distinguish the different contributions in contracture of the gastrocnemius and soleus muscles to the equinus deformity. In an office setting, it is often difficult to distinguish between the dynamic and static components of equinus deformity.

The final clinical evaluation is observation of the patient walking while barefoot. The velocity of walking can be calculated by timing the patient over a set distance. The Functional Ambulation Classification (**Table 2**) is a validated and clinically useful classification of walking ability.[31] It does not consider the need for bracing, shoe modifications, or upper extremity assistive devices, as many patients are unable to use such devices until their SEV deformity has been corrected.[3] The classification consists of 6 categories ranging from nonambulatory to normal walking.

Laboratory gait analysis and dynamic polyelectromyography have led to a better understanding of the etiology of equinovarus deformity. Such testing is also important to supplement a comprehensive physical examination to identify the specific muscle groups that are spastic and contribute to the deformity, and thereby guide treatment. Fuller and colleagues[23] performed a prospective study documenting that gait analysis resulted in a refinement of surgical planning in 64% of patients. The experience of the surgeon did not affect the impact of the gait analysis. With dynamic electromyography studies, Perry and colleagues[10] have demonstrated that, when varus deformity is observed in stroke patients, the tibialis anterior muscle is active during 80% of the swing phase and during the entire stance phase. Additionally, the activity of the posterior tibial muscle is variable, and the activity of the FHL muscle may be of critical importance in very spastic feet because toe flexors contribute to ankle plantarflexion. In patients who have had a stroke or traumatic brain injury, the tibialis posterior is less commonly a contributor to varus deformity.

An improved understanding of the complex causes of SEV deformity has resulted in the refinement and evolution the surgical procedures used to correct SEV deformity. For instance, as the SPLATT procedure has evolved, additional procedures have been included at the time of index surgery in order to optimize both the achievement and maintenance of a plantigrade foot and to maintain strength. Spasticity of the EHL muscle and resulting hyperextension deformity of the hallux are countered by an EHL transfer to the mid dorsum of the foot; this also provides an additional dorsiflexion force for the ankle. Patients require lifelong muscle balance of multiple muscle groups. As a result, the SPLATT procedure has become routinely combined with procedures such as Achilles tendon lengthening, posterior tibialis lengthening, and assorted transfers and releases of intrinsic and extrinsic foot flexor and extensor tendons.

SURGICAL TECHNIQUES
Correction of Equinus Deformity

It is difficult to distinguish between the relative contribution of dynamic spasticity and static contracture of the gastrocnemius, soleus, and Achilles to the equinus deformity. For this reason, the patient should be examined while awake and then reexamined while under anesthesia. If the equinus corrects under general anesthesia, the deformity is primarily dynamic (spastic). A proximal lengthening of the gastrocnemius and soleus muscles should be performed. Proximal lengthening saves more muscle strength. Intramuscular lengthening also preserves the elastic recoil provided by the Achilles tendon, which aids in push-off. A common mistake is to misinterpret correction of equinus deformity under anesthesia as a contraindication to surgical correction. A dynamic deformity requires alteration of the muscle imbalance caused by overactivity of the calf muscles. If the equinus deformity persists under anesthesia, there is a significant static contracture. In this situation the Achilles tendon needs lengthening to correct the deformity. Both procedures are described.

Achilles tendon lengthening (Hoke lengthening)

With Achilles tendon lengthening (Hoke lengthening) the foot is held in a maximally dorsiflexed position by the surgical assistant. A Number 11 scalpel blade is placed into the center of the Achilles tendon through a longitudinal stab incision, and then rotated 90° to perform the hemitransection cuts. Three percutaneous hemitransection cuts are made in a staggered fashion in the Achilles tendon, allowing the fibers to slide (**Fig. 4**). The most distal incision is made first just proximal to the insertion of the Achilles tendon. The second incision is made at the proximal extent of the Achilles tendon. A third incision is made halfway between the proximal and distal incisions. The staggered placement of the incisions ensures that there is sufficient overlap in the remaining tendon structure to prevent complete rupture.

After the cuts are made, the foot should be gently pressed into dorsiflexion, allowing the tendon fibers to slide. Care should be taken not to fully transect the tendon when making the cuts or to push with such force after hemitransection that an iatrogenic Achilles tendon rupture occurs. If complete transaction or rupture occurs, management options include primary suture repair of the Achilles tendon, as well as transfer of the FHL or FDL to the calcaneus. Secondary healing in cast immobilization is not recommended because this requires immobilization of the foot in equinus position and would defeat the purpose of the surgery.

If a varus deformity is present, the proximal and distal cuts in the tendon are made in the medial half of the tendon, and the center cut is made in the lateral half of the tendon. If a valgus deformity is present (rare), the proximal and distal cuts are made laterally, and the central cut is made medially.

Proximal lengthening of the gastrocnemius and soleus muscles

With proximal lengthening of the gastrocnemius and soleus muscles, a 5-cm incision is made over the medial leg at the mid portion of the gastrocnemius muscle belly. Dissection is carried through the subcutaneous tissue, and fascia is opened longitudinally. The plane between the gastrocnemius and soleus muscle bellies is developed

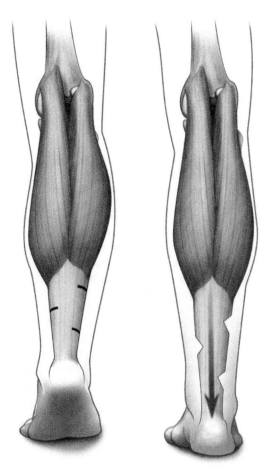

Fig. 4. The Hoke triple hemisection technique for lengthening of the Achilles tendon.

with blunt dissection. The tendons of gastrocnemius and soleus muscles are lengthened by transecting the tendons overlying the muscle bellies. The foot is gently pushed into dorsiflexion to allow the tendons to slide on the muscles.

Correction of Claw Toe Deformity

Flexion of the great toe results from overactivity of the FHL and flexor hallucis brevis muscles. The lesser toes also assume a position of marked flexion secondary to overactivity of the FDL and flexor digitorum brevis muscles. This is easily seen when the patient is standing. The FHL and FDL also contribute to the equinus deformity. The toe flexion increases when the foot is brought into a neutral plantigrade position, after correction of the equinus deformity. The claw toe deformity must therefore be corrected at the same time.

In the past, only the FHL and FDL tendons were released. This was done through the medial foot incision used to release the tibialis anterior tendon for the SPLATT. Commonly the toe flexion deformity persisted after surgery secondary to spasticity in the flexor hallucis brevis and flexor digitorum brevis muscles. Surgeons now routinely release all of the toe flexor tendons.[32]

A 1-cm longitudinal incision is made on the plantar aspect of the foot at the base of each of the five toes just proximal to the metatarsal-phalangeal joint. The incision is carried down through the subcutaneous tissue and fascia. Each toe is then dorsiflexed maximally to place the flexor tendons on tension. The scalpel is then used to transect the tendons transversely. The blade should be placed so it passes deep to the flexor tendons and contacts bone. This avoids inadvertent horizontal cuts in the skin. A horizontal incision is not performed because it leads to skin gapping after release of the flexor tendons.

Correction of Calf Weakness

A common misconception is that spastic muscles are "too strong." Muscle overactivity, the inability of a muscle to relax, or its exaggerated response to a quick stretch stimulus should not be interpreted as strength. Paresis is a prominent feature of UMNS. Spastic muscles are inherently weak muscles. The most common indication for use of an ankle-foot orthosis after SEV surgery is calf weakness. Lengthening of the Achilles tendon or fractional lengthening of the proximal gastrocnemius and soleus muscles further compromises the plantarflexion strength of patients with UMNS. Transfer of the FDL to the calcaneus has been shown to augment calf strength and decrease the need for bracing with ambulation after surgery.[33] Seventy percent of patients having an FDL to calcaneus transfer achieve ankle-foot orthosis (AFO)–free ambulation versus 30% of patients who realize AFO-free ambulation without FDL transfer.

A 4-cm incision is made on the medial border of the foot parallel and dorsal to the abductor hallucis. The incision is carried down through the subcutaneous tissues and fat. The abductor hallucis is then reflected plantarly to expose the master knot of Henry (**Fig. 5**). Care should be taken at the proximal aspect of the incision, as bleeding can be encountered where the medial and lateral plantar arteries branch off the posterior tibial artery. The FHL and FDL tendons are then dissected free and individually identified. A hemostat is used to isolate the FDL tendon. The tendon is then transected.

It is technically easier to identify and isolate the FDL tendon in the foot before distal release of the toe flexor tendons for correction of the claw toe deformity.

Next, a 3-cm longitudinal incision is made posterior to the medial malleolus. Care is taken to avoid the neurovascular bundle immediately posterior to the FDL tendon. The FDL is identified, and the distal cut end of the tendon is delivered proximally using a hemostat. A lasso suture of 1-0 Vicryl is placed in the distal cut end of the FDL tendon.

A 1-cm incision is then made over the medial calcaneus. A hemostat is used to bluntly dissect down to the calcaneus. A 5-mm drill is used to create a bony tunnel through the calcaneus medially to laterally. The skin over the lateral surface of the calcaneus is left intact. The FDL tendon is passed subcutaneously from the incision posterior to the medial malleolus to the medial calcaneal incision. To aid in the insertion of the tendon into the calcaneus, a meniscal needle is passed through the bony tunnel in the calcaneus from medial to lateral. The sharp end of the meniscal needle should protrude through the skin on the lateral aspect of the hindfoot. The free end of the suture attached to the FDL tendon is then passed through the bony tunnel in the calcaneus, followed by the tendon from medial to lateral using the meniscal needle. The suture is pulled through the skin on the lateral side.

Traction is placed on the suture to pull the FDL tendon into the calcaneal tunnel. Usually a distinct pop sensation is felt when this occurs. It is critical to ensure (through direct visualization) that the tendon has been completely passed into the bony tunnel of the calcaneus and is not protruding out of the tunnel (or has not become folded

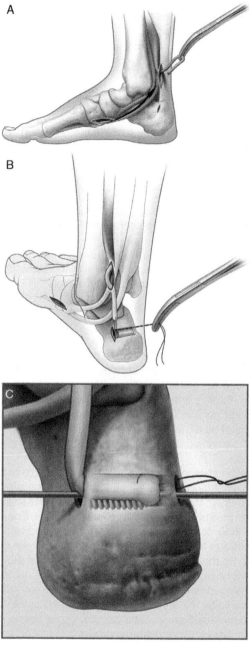

Fig. 5. The transfer of the FDL tendon to the calcaneus. (*A*) Harvesting of the FDL tendon. (*B*) Passing the FDL tendon into the calcaneal tunnel. (*C*) Fixation of the FDL tendon in the calcaneus using an interference screw.

over itself). To aid in proper passage of the tendon into the tunnel, a small forceps can be used to guide the tendon into the medial aspect of the tunnel.

Next, a Steinman pin is placed through the bony tunnel from the medial side of the heel to act as a guide wire. The foot is then placed in neutral dorsiflexion while tensioning the FDL, and a 7-mm by 20-mm bioabsorbable interference screw is passed over the guide wire.[34,35] Care should be taken to avoid plantarflexion when securing the tendon within the tunnel, as this will result in recurrent equinus deformity. The screw is advanced until it is seated completely within the bone, securing the FDL tendon within the calcaneus. The 7-mm interference screw creates a tight fit within the 5-mm bone tunnel. The suture protruding through the lateral aspect of the skin is then cut at the level of the skin.

Correction of Varus Deformity

The varus component of the equinovarus foot most commonly results from overactivity of the tibialis anterior muscle. A split anterior tibialis tendon transfer allows for one-half of the tendon to be transferred laterally to the cuboid and is usually sufficient to balance the varus force that stems from the medial half of the tendon. In a small percentage of patients, the varus deformity can also be accentuated by spasticity of the tibialis posterior muscle, which causes heel varus. This is corrected through a myotendinous lengthening of the tibialis posterior muscle.

Split anterior tibialis tendon transfer

With split anterior tibialis tendon transfer, a 3-cm longitudinal incision is made on the medial foot directly overlying the insertion of the anterior tibialis tendon. The fascia over the tendon is split to expose the tendon. A hemostat is placed under the tendon just proximal to its insertion. A Number 15 scalpel blade is placed directly in the center of the tendon and carried distally, splitting the tendon longitudinally into equal-diameter halves (**Fig. 6**). It is important that the tendon is divided equally to avoid rupture of either tendon portion. When the scalpel has reached the distal end of the tendon, the blade should be turned 90°, and the tendon should be transected laterally. A lasso suture of 1-0 Vicryl is then placed on the distal end of the tendon to facilitate passage of the tendon.

Next a 3-cm longitudinal incision is made over the anterior aspect of the distal third of the leg 10 cm proximal to the ankle joint and on the lateral side of the tibial crest. The incision is carried down through the subcutaneous tissues to expose the proximal aspect of the anterior tibialis muscle with its overlying fascia. The fascia is then split. A long twisted wire loop or other tendon passer is then passed from the proximal incision under the fascia to the medial foot incision. The suture in the distal end of the anterior tibialis tendon is then passed through the open end of the wire loop. The wire loop is pulled proximally, bringing the free end of the suture out through the anterior incision. The suture is used to deliver the lateral limb of the tendon proximally. As the tendon is pulled proximally, the anterior tibialis tendon splits into equal halves.

The next step is to make a 1-cm incision over the lateral border of the foot, directly over the cuboid bone. The extensor digitorum brevis is identified and reflected toward the dorsum of the foot to expose the lateral surface of the cuboid. A 5-mm drill is used to create a tunnel through the cuboid, directed medially. Bony tunnels, which are perpendicular to the surface of the bone, result in a stronger construct. There is less chance of a fracture in osteoporotic bone, the mechanical advantage of the transferred tendon is enhanced, and the pull-out strength of the interference screw is improved. With the advent of interference screws, the need to create a bony bridge/tunnel with intersecting drill holes has been obviated.

A   B

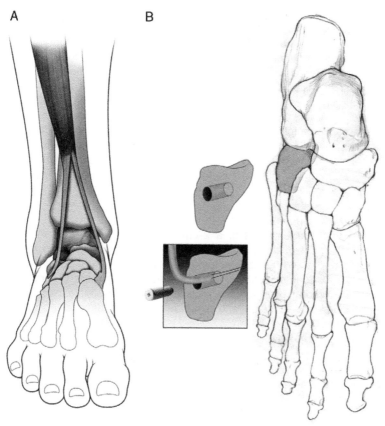

Fig. 6. The SPLATT. (*A*) The completed SPLATT transfer. (*B*) The tunnel in the cuboid bone for the lateral arm of the tibialis anterior tendon.

Long forceps are passed subcutaneously from the lateral foot incision to the anterior leg incision. The forceps are passed beneath the extensor brevis muscle belly to provide improved soft-tissue coverage distally. The lateral limb of the anterior tibialis tendon is then pulled distally to the lateral foot incision.

A meniscal needle is then passed through the cuboid tunnel with the sharp end of the needle exiting through the medial skin. The free end of the suture attached to the anterior tibialis tendon is next passed through the bony tunnel in the cuboid, followed by the tendon using the meniscal needle. The free end of the suture should be pulled until the foot is in a neutral position and the varus deformity has been corrected.

A Kirschner wire or Steinman pin is then placed into the bony tunnel with the tendon to act as a guide wire. A 7-mm diameter bioabsorbable interference screw is passed over the guide wire. The screw is advanced until it is seated completely within the bone, securing the anterior tibialis tendon within the cuboid. There should be no slack on the limb of the tendon that is attached to the cuboid, and the foot should rest in a balanced position. The suture protruding through the medial aspect of the skin is then cut at the level of the skin. Confirmation should be made at this point of the neutral position of the foot. With osteoporotic bone, there is the theoretical risk of screw pull-out. If this occurs, a new tunnel may be considered versus attachment of the harvested tendon to the peroneal brevis tendon.

It is important to tension the transferred tendon limbs with the foot in the neutral position. With this procedure, both limbs of the tibialis anterior are equally tensioned. The use of interference screws to secure the tendons in the bony tunnels makes tensioning much easier. Earlier techniques passed the lateral arm of the tibialis anterior through a dorsal-to-plantar tunnel in the cuboid and then sewed the tendon back on itself. This technique made tensioning in a balanced position more difficult, and fracture of the cuboid was more common. Overtensioning of the lateral limb to create a more powerful lateral pull may result in slackness in the medial limb, and it is not necessary to overcorrect the varus deformity. When static balance of tendon pull is obtained intraoperatively, dynamic balance of the foot can be expected over the long term.

Tibialis posterior lengthening

With tibialis posterior lengthening, a 2-cm longitudinal incision is made on the posteromedial aspect of the distal third of the leg and carried down through the subcutaneous tissue and fascia. The fascia overlying the tibialis posterior tendon is split, and the tendon is identified and isolated. The muscle is lengthened by transecting the tendon overlying the muscle belly. Care should be taken not to transect the distal tendon, as a planovalgus deformity can develop.

Correction of Hallux Hyperextension and Forefoot Varus

Often the contribution of the EHL to varus is not appreciated when observing the patient standing and walking. In an equinovarus deformity, patients may develop great toe pain owing to pressure of the hallux against the shoe from EHL spasticity. Correction of the painful hallux while improving the strength and balance of forefoot dorsiflexion can be accomplished by transfer of the EHL tendon to the mid dorsum of the foot (**Fig. 7**). To avoid hallux droop, the distal EHL tendon is sutured to the extensor digitorum brevis or the medial aspect of the tibialis anterior to create a tenodesis.

A 2-cm longitudinal incision is made over the lateral border of the EHL tendon on the dorsum of the foot. The tendon sheath is opened, and the EHL tendon is isolated. Dissection is then carried deep onto the bony surface of the foot laterally to fully expose the middle cuneiform bone. Care is taken to avoid the neurovascular bundle, which lies deep and lateral to the EHL tendon.

The EHL tendon is transected distally. A lasso suture of 1-0 Vicryl is then placed in the distal cut end of the tendon. A 5-mm drill bit is used to drill a bony tunnel from dorsal to plantar through the middle cuneiform. The tunnel is directed posteriorly to improve pull-out strength. A meniscal needle is placed in the tunnel drilled in the middle cuneiform, with the sharp end of the needle exiting through the plantar skin. As previously described, a combination of the meniscal needle and Steinman pin is used to pass the tendon and then secure it in place within the middle cuneiform with a 7-mm diameter bioabsorbable interference screw. The foot is held in a neutral position as this is performed.

AFTER-CARE

At the conclusion of each of the previous procedures, the tourniquet is deflated, hemostasis obtained, and the wounds closed. On completion of the procedure and dressing application, the patient is placed in a short-leg weight-bearing cast. The cast should be well padded and must maintain the foot in the corrected position. It is

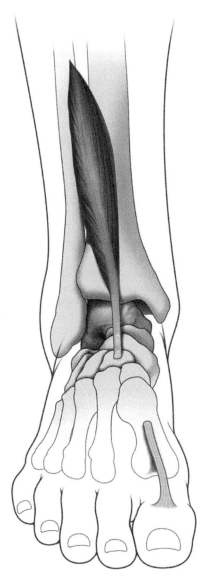

Fig. 7. The transfer of the EHL tendon to the middle cuneiform bone.

critical for the patient to be fully under anesthesia during the placement of the cast so that the foot does not drift back into equinovarus position as the patient awakens. Pain enhances spasticity. In addition to adequate pain management, drug therapy is needed for the first week after surgery to control the spasticity. Diazepam is an effective medication for the short-term control of muscle tone. If the patient is already using antispasticity medication, the dosage can be increased as tolerated. If the patient has an intrathecal baclofen pump, the infusion dosage can be increased.

The patient is allowed immediate full weight-bearing ambulation and transfers in the cast. The cast is changed 2 weeks after surgery and continued for a total of

6 weeks. The patient is then placed in a rigid AFO for an additional 6 weeks to allow full healing of the transferred and lengthened tendons. The AFO is worn 24 hours per day.

Twelve weeks after surgery the patient can begin active strengthening exercises and attempt to wean from dependence on the AFO. The therapist, patient, and family should be cautioned to avoid passive plantarflexion of the foot as this could result in recurrent equinus.

COMPLICATIONS

Complications are uncommon. Complications can be divided between those associated with general operative management and those specific to the various tendon transfer procedures. General risks include wound healing complications and superficial soft-tissue infection. Deep venous thrombosis with postoperative immobilization is infrequent. Other potential complications include failure of fixation and rupture of transferred tendon constructs. Interference screw pull-out may be observed infrequently.[35] Pull-outs most often occur with the EHL transfer. Directing the tunnel posteriorly in the middle cuneiform bone reduces this problem.

Recurrence of deformity is rare and can be corrected with further surgery if needed. Recurrence is lessened by performing all needed tendon transfers and lengthenings in a single surgery. The patient and family must be strongly advised that the goal of surgery is to obtain a plantigrade foot and that future independence from an AFO is not achieved in all patients.

SUMMARY

The surgical correction of SEV foot and ankle deformity is well-established and yields excellent clinical results. Ambulation, transfers, functional improvements, muscle strengthening, and progression from assistive aids have all been documented in the literature. These results lead to an overall improvement in quality of life for the patient and their caretakers. Surgery itself may be a more cost-effective method of treatment when compared with a protracted course of nonoperative treatment.

REFERENCES

1. Mayer NH, Herman RM. Positive signs and consequences of an upper motor neuron syndrome. In: Brashear A, Mayer NH, editors. Spasticity and other forms of muscle overactivity in the upper motor neuron syndrome: etiology, evaluation, management and the role of botulinum toxin. New York (NY): WeMove.org; 2008. p.11–26.
2. Pinzur MS, Sherman R, DiMonte-Levine P, et al. Adult-onset hemiplegia: changes in gait after muscle-balancing procedures to correct the equinus deformity. J Bone Joint Surg [Am] 1986;68:1249–57.
3. Keenan MA, Creighton J, Garland DE, et al. Surgical correction of spastic equinovarus deformity in the adult head trauma patient. Foot Ankle 1984;5:35–41.
4. Keenan MA, Mayer NH, Esquenazi A, et al. A neuro-orthopaedic approach to the management of common patterns of upper motoneuron dysfunction after brain injury. Journal of Neuro Rehabilitation 1999;12:119–43.
5. Keenan MAE, Lee G. Orthopaedic management of lower extremity dysfunction following stroke or brain injury. In: Chapman M, editor. Chapman's operative orthopaedics. Philadelphia: Lippincott Williams and Wilkins; 2001. p. 3201–43.
6. Lawrence SJ, Botte MJ. Management of the adult, spastic, equinovarus foot deformity. Foot Ankle Int 1994;15:340–6.
7. Banks HH. The management of spastic deformities of the foot and ankle. Clin Orthop Relat Res 1977;122:70–6.

8. Keenan MA, Perry J, Jordan C. Factors affecting balance and ambulation following stroke. Clin Orthop Relat Res 1984;182:165–71.
9. Reddy S, Kusuma S, Hosalkar H, et al. Surgery can reduce the nonoperative care associated with an equinovarus foot deformity. Clin Orthop Relat Res 2008;466: 1683–7.
10. Perry J, Waters R, Perrin T. Electromyographic analysis of equinovarus following stroke. Clin Orthop Relat Res 1978;131:4753.
11. Waters RL, Frazier J, Garland DE, et al. Electromyographic gait analysis before and after operative treatment for hemiplegic equinus and equinovarus deformity. J Bone Joint Surg 1982;64:284–8.
12. Holden MK, Gill KM, Magliozzi MR. Gait assessment for neurologically impaired patients. Standards for outcome assessment. Phys Ther 1986;66:1530–9.
13. Keenan MA. Surgical decision making for residual limb deformities following traumatic brain injury. Orthop Rev 1988;17:1185–92.
14. Edwards P, Hsu J. SPLATT combined with tendo Achilles lengthening for spastic equinovarus in adults: results and predictors of surgical outcome. Foot Ankle 1993; 14:335–8.
15. Hoffer MM, Reiswig JA, Garret AM, et al. The split anterior tibial tendon transfer in the treatment of spastic varus hindfoot in childhood. Orthop Clin North Am 1974;5:31–8.
16. Lemperg R, Hagberg B, Lundberg A. Achilles tenoplasty for correction of equinus deformity in spastic syndromes of cerebral palsy. Acta Orthop Scand 1969;40: 507–19.
17. Roper BA, Williams A, King JB. The surgical treatment of equinovarus deformity in adults with spasticity. J Bone Joint Surg [Br] 1978;60-B:533–5.
18. Ono K, Hiroshima K, Tada K, et al. Anterior transfer of the toe flexors for equinovarus deformity of the foot. Int Orthop 1980;4:225–9.
19. Barnes MJ, Herring JA. Combined split anterior tibial-tendon transfer and intramuscular lengthening of the posterior tibial tendon. Results in patients who have a varus deformity of the foot due to spastic cerebral palsy. J Bone Joint Surg [Am] 1991;73: 734–8.
20. Dunkerley DR. The role of surgery in rehabilitation. Int Rehabil Med 1985;7:39–40.
21. Jordan C. Current status of functional lower extremity surgery in adult spastic patients. Clin Orthop Relat Res 1988;233:102–9.
22. Perry J. Contractures. A historical perspective. Clin Orthop Relat Res 1987;219:8–14.
23. Fuller DA, Keenan MAE, Esquenazi A, et al. The impact of instrumented gait analysis on surgical planning: treatment of spastic equinovarus deformity of the foot and ankle. Foot Ankle Int 2002;23(8):738–43.
24. Namdari S, Park M, Baldwin K, et al. Correcting spastic equinovarus post-cerebrovascular accident: Do age, sex, and timing matter? Foot Ankle Int 2009;30(10):923–7.
25. Walshe FMR. On certain tonic or postural reflexes in hemiplegia, with special reference to the so-called "associated movements." Brain 1923;46:1–37.
26. Ashworth B. Preliminary trial of carisoprodol in multiple sclerosis. Practitioner 1964: 192:540–2.
27. Lee KC, Carson L, Kinnin E, et al. The Ashworth scale: a reliable and reproducible method of measuring spasticity. J Neurol Rehabil 1989;3:205–9.
28. Bohannon RW, Smith MB. Interrater reliability of modified Ashworth scale of muscle spasticity. Phys Ther 1987;67(2):206–7.
29. Silfverskiold N. Reduction of the uncrossed two-joints muscles of the leg to one-joint muscles in spastic conditions. Acta Chir Scand 1924;56:315–30.
30. DiGiovanni CW, Kuo R, Tejwani N, et al. Isolated gastrocnemius tightness. J Bone Joint Surg [Am] 2002;84-A:962–70.

31. Viosca E, Martinez JL, Almagro PL, et al. Proposal and validation of a new functional ambulation classification scale for clinical use. Arch Phys Med Rehabil 2005;86: 1234–8.
32. Keenan MA, Gorai AP, Smith CW, et al. Intrinsic toe flexion deformity following correction of spastic equinovarus deformity in adults. Foot Ankle 1987;7:333–7.
33. Keenan MA, Lee GA, Tuckman AS, et al. Improving calf muscle strength in patients with spastic equinovarus deformity by transfer of the long toe flexors to the Os calcis. J Head Trauma Rehabil 1999;14:163–75.
34. Fuller DA, McCarthy JJ, Keenan MA. The use of the absorbable interference screw for a split anterior tibial tendon (SPLATT) transfer procedure. Orthopedics 2004;27: 372–4.
35. Hosalkar H, Goebel J, Reddy S, et al. Fixation techniques for split anterior tibialis transfer in spastic equinovarus feet. Clin Orthop Relat Res 2008;466:2500–6.

Index

Note: Page numbers of article titles are in **boldface** type.

A

Abductor hallucis (ABH) tendon transfer, for hallux varus, technique for, 458–462
    bone tunnels and course diagram in, 458, 460
    capsulotomy and release in, 452
    ideal position in, 458, 460
    proximal release in, 458–459
Achilles tendon, contracture of, in equinovalgus foot, 489–490, 492
  in cavovarus foot, 436
Achilles tendon lengthening, for spastic equinovarus foot deformity, 499, 504–505
Hoke procedure for, 491–492
  in anterior tibialis tendon transfer, for equinovarus deformity, in adults, 412
  in bridle procedure, authors' preferences for, 423–424
    for equinovarus deformity, in adults, 411
  in posterior tibial tendon transfer, for equinovarus deformity, in adults, 407
  percutaneous, for equinovalgus foot, 491–492
    for foot drop, 377
    for motor imbalance, 380
    for spasticity, 380–381
Actin–myosin overlap, in muscle length vs. tension relationship, 390–391
Adult flexible cavovarus deformity, tendon transfers for, **435–450**. See also *Cavovarus foot.*
Ambulation Scale, Functional, in spastic equinovarus foot deformity evaluation, 503
Amplitude, appropriate, in tendon transfers, 387–388
Anchoring. See *Bone anchor; Suture anchor fixation; Tendon anchoring.*
Aneurysm needle, in extensor digitorum brevis tendon transfer, for forefoot deformities, 483–484
Ankle deformity, valgus, with paralytic equinovalgus deformity, 490–491
  varus, with equinovarus deformity, in adults, 407
Ankle dorsiflexion, in spastic equinovarus foot deformity evaluation, 502–503
Ankle foot orthosis (AFO), postoperative, for spastic equinovarus foot deformity, 512
    calf weakness as indication, 506
    for tendon transfers, 378, 413
  tendon transfers vs., for foot drop, 376–377
    for motor imbalance, 380
    for spastic equinovarus, 380
Anterior compartment muscle debridement, bridle procedure following, 420–421, 423
    fascia repair of, operative, 430, 432
Anterior tibial tendon sheath, in physiologic transfer, of peroneal tendons, for equinovalgus deformity, 493
Anterior tibialis tendon, in bridle procedure, 419–421, 426–427, 430

Foot Ankle Clin N Am 16 (2011) 515–536
doi:S1083-7515(11)00070-2
1083-7515/11/$ – see front matter © 2011 Elsevier Inc. All rights reserved.

foot.theclinics.com

M

Printed and bound by CPI Group (UK) Ltd, Croydon, CR0 4YY

03/10/2024

01040449-0013